Developmental Programming in Livestock Production

Editors

RICK N. FUNSTON
J. TRAVIS MULLINIKS

VETERINARY CLINICS
OF NORTH AMERICA:
FOOD ANIMAL PRACTICE

www.vetfood.theclinics.com

Consulting Editor
ROBERT A. SMITH

July 2019 • Volume 35 • Number 2

ELSEVIER

1600 John F. Kennedy Boulevard ● Suite 1800 ● Philadelphia, Pennsylvania, 19103-2899

http://www.vetfood.theclinics.com

**VETERINARY CLINICS OF NORTH AMERICA: FOOD ANIMAL PRACTICE Volume 35, Number 2
July 2019 ISSN 0749-0720, ISBN-13: 978-0-323-67884-1**

Editor: Colleen Dietzler
Developmental Editor: Meredith Madeira

Veterinary Clinics of North America: Food Animal Practice (ISSN 0749-0720) is published in March, July, and November by Elsevier Inc., 360 Park Avenue South, New York, NY 10010-1710. Subscription prices are $256.00 per year (domestic individuals), $434.00 per year (domestic institutions), $100.00 per year (domestic students/residents), $283.00 per year (Canadian individuals), $572.00 per year (Canadian institutions), $335.00 per year (international individuals), $572.00 per year (international institutions), and $165.00 per year (international and Canadian students/residents). To receive student/resident rate, orders must be accompanied by name of affiliated institution, date of term, and the signature of program/residency coordinator on institution letterhead. *Clinics* subscription prices. All prices are subject to change without notice. **POSTMASTER:** Send address changes to *Veterinary Clinics of North America: Food Animal Practice*, Elsevier Health Sciences Division, Subscription Customer Service, 3251 Riverport Lane, Maryland Heights, MO 63043. Customer Service (orders, claims, online, change of address): Elsevier Health Sciences Division, Subscription **Customer Service, 3251 Riverport Lane, Maryland Heights, MO 63043. Tel: 1-800-654-2452 (U.S. and Canada); 314-447-8871 (ouside U.S. and Canada). Fax: 314-447-8029. E-mail: journalscustomerservice-usa@elsevier.com (for print support); journalsonlinesupport-usa@elsevier.com (for online support).**

Reprints. For copies of 100 or more, of articles in this publication, please contact the Commercial Reprints Department, Elsevier Inc., 360 Park Avenue South, New York, NY 10010-1710. Tel.: 212-633-3874; Fax: 212-633-3820; E-mail: reprints@elsevier.com.

Veterinary Clinics of North America: Food Animal Practice is covered in *Current Contents/Agriculture, Biology and Environmental Sciences, MEDLINE/PubMed (Index Medicus), and Excerpta Medica.*

Contributors

CONSULTING EDITOR

ROBERT A. SMITH, DVM, MS
Diplomate, American Board of Veterinary Practitioners; Veterinary Research and Consulting Services, LLC, Greeley, Colorado, USA

EDITORS

RICK N. FUNSTON, PhD
Reproductive Physiologist, University of Nebraska, West Central Research and Extension Center, North Platte, Nebraska, USA

J. TRAVIS MULLINIKS, PhD
Range Cattle Nutritionist, Beef Production Systems, University of Nebraska, West Central Research and Extension Center, North Platte, Nebraska, USA

AUTHORS

ALAN W. BELL, PhD
Emeritus Professor, Department of Animal Science, Cornell University, Ithaca, New York, USA

PAWEL P. BOROWICZ, DVM, PhD
Research Assistant Professor, Advanced Imaging and Microscopy Core Lab, Department of Animal Sciences, Center for Nutrition and Pregnancy, North Dakota State University, Fargo, North Dakota, USA

DEVIN BROADHEAD, BS
Technologist I, Agricultural Economics, University of Nebraska, West Central Research and Extension Center, North Platte, Nebraska, USA

JOEL S. CATON, PhD
Professor, Department of Animal Sciences, Center for Nutrition and Pregnancy, North Dakota State University, Fargo, North Dakota, USA

REINALDO F. COOKE, PhD
Associate Professor, Department of Animal Science, Texas A&M University, College Station, Texas, USA

K.J. COPPING, PhD
Robinson Research Institute, University of Adelaide, South Australia, Australia

MATTHEW S. CROUSE, MS
USDA-NIFA-AFRI Predoctoral Research Fellow, Department of Animal Sciences, Center for Nutrition and Pregnancy, North Dakota State University, Fargo, North Dakota, USA

ROBERT A. CUSHMAN, PhD
Lead Scientist and Research Physiologist, Nutrition and Environmental Management
Research Unit, USDA, ARS, U.S. Meat Animal Research Center, Clay Center, Nebraska,
USA

GEOFFREY E. DAHL, PhD
Harriet B. Weeks Professor, Department of Animal Sciences, Institute of Food and
Agricultural Sciences, University of Florida, Gainesville, Florida, USA

CARL R. DAHLEN, PhD
Associate Professor, Department of Animal Sciences, Center for Nutrition and Pregnancy,
North Dakota State University, Fargo, North Dakota, USA

CALLUM G. DONNELLY, BVSc (Hons 1), DACT
Chief Resident, Department of Medicine and Epidemiology, School of Veterinary
Medicine, University of California, Davis, Davis, California, USA

AHMED ELOLIMY, MS
Mammalian NutriPhysioGenomics, Department of Animal Sciences, Division of Nutritional
Sciences, University of Illinois, Urbana, Illinois, USA

RICK N. FUNSTON, PhD
Reproductive Physiologist, University of Nebraska, West Central Research and Extension
Center, North Platte, Nebraska, USA

PAUL L. GREENWOOD, PhD
Senior Principal Research Scientist, NSW Department of Primary Industries, Armidale
Livestock Industries Centre, University of New England, Armidale, New South Wales,
Australia

EL HAMIDI HAY, PhD
USDA, ARS, Fort Keogh Livestock and Range Research Laboratory, Miles City, Montana,
USA

J. HERNANDEZ-MEDRANO, DVM, MSc, PhD
Academic Division of Child Health, Obstetrics and Gynaecology, School of Medicine,
Queen's Medical Centre, The University of Nottingham, Nottingham, United Kingdom

JIMENA LAPORTA, PhD
Assistant Professor, Department of Animal Sciences, Institute of Food and Agricultural
Sciences, University of Florida, Gainesville, Florida, USA

YAHAN LI, BS, MS
Division of Animal Sciences, University of Missouri, Columbia, Missouri, USA

YUSHENG LIANG, MS
Mammalian NutriPhysioGenomics, Department of Animal Sciences, Division of Nutritional
Sciences, University of Illinois, Urbana, Illinois, USA

JUAN J. LOOR, PhD
Mammalian NutriPhysioGenomics, Department of Animal Sciences, Division of Nutritional
Sciences, University of Illinois, Urbana, Illinois, USA

G. MIGUEL-PACHECO, DVM, MSc, PhD
School of Veterinary and Medical Science, University of Nottingham, Sutton Bonington,
United Kingdom

J. TRAVIS MULLINIKS, PhD
Range Cattle Nutritionist, Beef Production Systems, University of Nebraska, West Central Research and Extension Center, North Platte, Nebraska, USA

GEORGE A. PERRY, PhD
Professor, Department of Animal Science, South Dakota State University, Brookings, South Dakota, USA

V.E.A. PERRY, PhD
Robinson Research Institute, University of Adelaide, South Australia, Australia

ROBERT J. POSONT, HBSC, MS
Stress Physiology Graduate Student, Department of Animal Science, University of Nebraska–Lincoln, Lincoln, Nebraska, USA

LAWRENCE P. REYNOLDS, PhD
University Distinguished Professor, Department of Animal Sciences, Center for Nutrition and Pregnancy, North Dakota State University, Fargo, North Dakota, USA

ROCÍO MELISSA RIVERA, BS, MS, PhD
Division of Animal Sciences, University of Missouri, Columbia, Missouri, USA

ANDREW J. ROBERTS, PhD
USDA, ARS, Fort Keogh Livestock and Range Research Laboratory, Miles City, Montana, USA

ERIC J. SCHOLLJEGERDES, PhD
Associate Professor, Department of Animal and Range Sciences, New Mexico State University, Las Cruces, New Mexico, USA

AMY L. SKIBIEL, PhD
Assistant Professor, Department of Animal Sciences, Institute of Food and Agricultural Sciences, University of Florida, Gainesville, Florida, USA

ADAM F. SUMMERS, PhD
Assistant Professor, Department of Animal and Range Sciences, New Mexico State University, Las Cruces, New Mexico, USA

MARIO VAILATI-RIBONI, MS
Mammalian NutriPhysioGenomics, Department of Animal Sciences, Division of Nutritional Sciences, University of Illinois, Urbana, Illinois, USA

ALISON K. WARD, PhD
Assistant Professor, Department of Animal Sciences, Center for Nutrition and Pregnancy, North Dakota State University, Fargo, North Dakota, USA

DUSTIN T. YATES, BS, MS, PhD
Assistant Professor of Stress Physiology, Department of Animal Science, University of Nebraska–Lincoln, Lincoln, Nebraska, USA

Contents

Maternal stressors that affect fetal development result in "developmental programming," which is associated with increased risk of various chronic pathologic conditions in the offspring, including metabolic syndrome; growth abnormalities; and reproductive, immune, behavioral, or cognitive dysfunction that can persist throughout their lifetime and even across subsequent generations. Developmental programming thus can lead to poor health, reduced longevity, and reduced productivity. Current research aims to develop management and therapeutic strategies to optimize fetal growth and development and thereby overcome the negative consequences of developmental programming, leading to improved health, longevity, and productivity of offspring.

In the context of physiologic responses that determine the growth, development, and health status of livestock, the role of epigenetics and the underlying cellular mechanisms it affects remain to be fully elucidated. Although recent work has provided evidence that maternal dietary energy level, carbohydrate type, or intestinal supply of methyl donors can elicit molecular changes in tissues of the embryo, fetus, or neonate, there are few data linking epigenetics with biochemical and physiologic outcomes. Therefore, efforts linking the epigenome with physiologic and developmental outcomes offer exciting opportunities for discoveries that can impact efficiency of nutrient use and well-being of livestock.

Large offspring syndrome (LOS) is a fetal overgrowth condition in bovines most often observed in offspring conceived with the use of assisted reproductive technologies (ART). Phenotypes observed in LOS include, overgrowth, enlarged tongues, umbilical hernias, muscle and skeleton malformations, abnormal organ growth and placental development. Although LOS cases have only been reported to be associated with ART, fetal overgrowth can occur spontaneously in cattle (S-LOS). S-LOS refers to oversized calves that are born at normal gestation lengths. ART-induced LOS has been characterized as an epigenetic syndrome, more specifically, a loss-of-imprinting condition. We propose that S-LOS is also a loss-of-imprinting condition.

Fetal stress induces developmental adaptations that result in intrauterine growth restriction (IUGR) and low birthweight. These adaptations reappropriate nutrients to the most essential tissues, which benefits fetal survival. The same adaptations are detrimental to growth efficiency and carcass value in livestock, however, because muscle is disproportionally targeted. IUGR adipocytes, liver tissues, and pancreatic β-cells also exhibit functional adaptations. Identifying mechanisms underlying adaptive changes is fundamental to improving outcomes and value in low birthweight livestock. The article outlines studies that have begun to identify stress-induced fetal adaptations affecting growth, metabolism, and differential nutrient utilization in IUGR-born animals.

The greatest loss in ruminant production systems occurs during the neonatal period. The maternal environment (nutrition and physiologic status) influences neonatal mortality and morbidity as it reportedly affects (a) Dystocia, both via increasing birth weight and placental dysfunction; (b) Neonatal thermoregulation, both via altering the amount of brown adipose tissue and its ability to function via effects upon the hypothalamic–pituitary–thyroid axis; (c) Modification of the developing immune system and its symbiotic nutrient sources; (d) Modification of maternal and neonatal behavior.

Maternal regulation of fetal development has consequences for growth and development of carcass tissues. Severely restricted fetal growth can reduce postnatal growth capacity, resulting in smaller-for-age animals that take longer to reach market weights but has little effect on feedlot efficiency or carcass and meat quality. Specific nutritional supplementation, particularly during later pregnancy, may limit fetal growth retardation and enhance postnatal growth capacity and carcass characteristics, and may improve development of intramuscular fat. Continued improvements in understanding developmental processes and their regulation will increase future capacity to improve growth, efficiency, carcasses, and meat quality through developmental programming.

Developmental programming became an area of interest to understand negative environmental impacts on progeny performance. Recently, the concept that we may be able to harness developmental programming to target animals to their niche in the production system has gained recognition. Female fertility is an area where developmental programming has been moderately successful; however, the mechanisms remain unclear. Although some studies have demonstrated differences in gonadal development and attainment of puberty in response to developmental programming, these have not translated to improved fertility. To improve response to developmental programming, it is critical to identify factors that contribute to inconsistencies across studies.

The concept of developmental programming was established using epidemiologic studies that investigated chronic illnesses in humans, such as coronary heart disease and hypertension. In livestock species, the impacts of developmental programming are important for production and welfare reasons and are used as research models for human and other animal species. Dams should be in adequate nutritional status to ensure optimal nutrient supply for fetal growth, including development of their immune system. Beef and dairy cows with insufficient nutrient intake during gestation produce calves with reduced immunity against diseases, such as scours, respiratory disease, and mastitis.

Heat stress during late gestation adversely impacts the developing calf. Calves that experience heat stress are born at a lower bodyweight and those deficits persist at least until puberty. In utero heat stress reduces passive transfer and calf survival. Late gestation heat stress programs a phenotype with lower milk yield, relative to herd mates born to cooled dams, in the first lactation and subsequent lactations.

Environmental influences resulting in epigenetic mediation of gene expression can affect multiple generations via direct effect (first generation); direct or maternally mediated effects on the fetus (second generation), or gonadal cell lines of the fetus (third generation) when pregnant animals are exposed to the stimuli; and through generational inheritance. The cumulative effects are rapid changes in phenotypic characteristics of the population when compared with rate of phenotypic change from genetic selection. With extensive data collection, significant potential exists to propagate desired characteristics in the livestock industry through epigenetic pathways.

Stimuli experienced in utero can have a lasting impact on livestock growth, reproduction, and performance. Variations in environment, production system, and management strategies lead to discrepancies in the literature regarding how specific treatments influence animal performance. Studies comparing the influence of maternal undernutrition to well-fed counterparts typically result in decreased productivity of offspring. Via adaptation to nutritional or environmental stressors, dams may develop mechanisms to ensure proper nutrient supply to the fetus. It appears nutrient deprivation must be severe for consistent results. Potential mechanisms for altered performance in grazing systems and overnutrition settings are discussed.

Developmental Programming in a Beef Production System

Devin Broadhead, J. Travis Mulliniks, and Rick N. Funston

Beef production is a complex system, in which cows are expected to perform in varied environmental conditions. In cattle, the most commonly reported developmental programming influence is nutrient restriction during the prenatal period due to climatic conditions affecting forage availability and quality. Recent research has demonstrated maternal or prepartum nutrition can affect more than just subsequent pregnancy rates. Studies in different species report how maternal nutrition influences progeny performance, health, and reproduction. Better understanding of developmental programming and nutritional management within different environments may advance cowherd efficiency.

VETERINARY CLINICS OF NORTH AMERICA: FOOD ANIMAL PRACTICE

SERIES OF RELATED INTEREST

Veterinary Clinics of North America: Exotic Animal Practice
Available: https://www.vetexotic.theclinics.com/

THE CLINICS ARE NOW AVAILABLE ONLINE!
Access your subscription at:
www.theclinics.com

VETERINARY CLINICS OF
NORTH AMERICA:
FOOD ANIMAL PRACTICE

FORTHCOMING ISSUES

November 2019
Ruminant Immunology
Christopher Chase, Editor

March 2020
Ruminant Parasitology
Ray M. Kaplan, Editor

July 2020
Toxicology
Steve Ensley, Editor

RECENT ISSUES

March 2019
How to to Dedicate Comfort, Health and
Productivity of Dairy Cattle
Nigel B. Cook, Editor

November 2018
Mastitis
Pamela L. Ruegg and
Christina S. Petersson-Wolfe, Editors

July 2018
Digestive Disease in Beef Cattle
Operations
Sammine R. Navarre and
Daniel U. Thomson, Editors

SERIES OF RELATED INTEREST

Veterinary Clinics of North America: Exotic Animal Practice
Available at: www.vetexotic.theclinics.com

Preface

Developmental Programming in Livestock Production

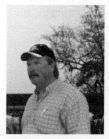 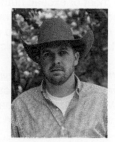

Rick N. Funston, PhD   J. Travis Mulliniks, PhD
Editors

The concept of fetal programming, also known as developmental programming, was first hypothesized using human epidemiologic data, where environmental stimulus in utero resulted in long-term development changes in growth and disease susceptibility in children from undernourished mothers during the Dutch famine. This concept is important due to the impact that maternal stimulus or insult at a critical period in fetal development has long-term effects on the offspring. While maternal nutrient delivery during pregnancy has been shown to program the growth and development of the fetus, both during pregnancy and later into adult life, it appears that maternal nutrition also programs the development of the placenta. While the timing and exact nutrients are not yet clearly delineated, it appears that different physiologic systems (ie, reproductive axis, muscle development) may be impacted at different time points during pregnancy.

Pasture- and range-based grazing systems vary tremendously across environments that differ in climate, topography, and forage production. This variation in environmental conditions contributes to the challenges of developing or targeting specific grazing and/or nutrient input systems. Environmental conditions and long-term management can impact how livestock respond to environmental stress and nutrient restriction. With environments and management practices, responses to developmental programming have been highly variable. Factors influencing fetal programming and the variation in response to fetal programming include age of the dam, number of fetuses, genetic potential, long-term management, and environmental stress. These factors play a role in programming the fetus for its future environment and available resources. Continual understanding of developmental processes and their regulation will increase future capacity to improve growth, efficiency, carcasses, and meat quality through developmental programming.

Vet Clin Food Anim 35 (2019) xiii–xiv
https://doi.org/10.1016/j.cvfa.2019.03.001
0749-0720/19/© 2019 Published by Elsevier Inc.

In recent years, livestock production has been challenged with balancing rising costs of production with output traits. Thus, beef production is faced with the question of how to optimize the utilization of feed resources to increase efficiency of beef production systems. Providing appropriate nutrition to cattle is the key to maintaining and improving beef production efficiency, as feed costs represent the largest portion of total production costs. Adequate nutrition programs are vital to optimize health and production in beef cattle production systems. However, efficiency and longevity may be reduced in beef herds due to managing to meet or exceed nutrient requirements during key physiologic periods allowing for reduced exposure to moderate stress. Cows that have been adapted and managed to reproduce in limited nutrient environments may have the ability to maintain normal fetal growth and development during periods of maternal nutrient restriction.

In this issue of *Veterinary Clinics of North America: Food Animal Practice*, we have invited authors to provide a comprehensive overview of developmental programming in livestock from conception to slaughter. We would like to thank each of the contributing authors for their time and effort in sharing their expertise for this issue.

Rick N. Funston, PhD
University of Nebraska
West Central Research and Extension Center
402 West State Farm Road
North Platte, NE 69101, USA

J. Travis Mulliniks, PhD
University of Nebraska
West Central Research and Extension Center
402 West State Farm Road
North Platte, NE 69101, USA

E-mail addresses:
rick.funston@unl.edu (R.N. Funston)
travis.mulliniks@unl.edu (J.T. Mulliniks)

Developmental Programming of Fetal Growth and Development

Lawrence P. Reynolds, PhD[a],*, Pawel P. Borowicz, DVM, PhD[b],
Joel S. Caton, PhD[a], Matthew S. Crouse, MS[a],
Carl R. Dahlen, PhD[a], Alison K. Ward, PhD[a]

KEYWORDS

- Fetus • Placenta • Growth • Development • Maternal stress
- Developmental programming • Postnatal health

KEY POINTS

- Stressors during pregnancy, including poor maternal diet, young or advanced maternal age, maternal or embryonic genetic background/breed/strain, environmental stress (eg, high environmental temperature, high altitude, exposure to environmental contaminants), assisted reproductive techniques (eg, in vitro fertilization, cloning, embryo transfer), or, in humans, lifestyle choices (eg, smoking, alcoholic consumption) can profoundly affect fetal growth and development.

- Altered fetal growth and development, in turn, often result in long-term changes in organ structure (eg, altered number of nephrons in the kidney, altered pancreatic islet number or size, altered myofiber number) or function, or both, resulting in increased risk of various chronic diseases (metabolic disorders, abnormal growth, reproductive dysfunction, immune dysfunction, behavioral and cognitive dysfunction, and so forth) in the offspring throughout their lifetime and perhaps even across subsequent generations.

- Recent studies suggest that despite the low metabolic demands of early pregnancy, the effects of stressors, such as poor maternal diet and assisted reproductive techniques (eg, in vitro fertilization), are "programmed" during the earliest stages of fetal growth and development.

- Research is currently aimed at developing management and therapeutic strategies to overcome the developmental programming effects of these various stressors, leading to improved health, longevity, and productivity of animals.

Disclosure: The authors have nothing to disclose.
[a] Department of Animal Sciences, Center for Nutrition and Pregnancy, North Dakota State University, NDSU Department 7630, Fargo, ND 58108-6050, USA; [b] Advanced Imaging and Microscopy Core Lab, Department of Animal Sciences, Center for Nutrition and Pregnancy, North Dakota State University, NDSU Department 7630, Fargo, ND 58108-6050, USA
* Corresponding author.
E-mail address: larry.reynolds@ndsu.edu

INTRODUCTION

Developmental programming, sometimes also known as fetal programming, refers to the concept that factors affecting fetal growth and development lead to long-term changes in organ structure (eg, altered number of nephrons in the kidney, altered pancreatic islet number or size, altered number of myofibers) or function, or both.[1–9] Such alterations, in turn, are associated with increased risk of various chronic pathologic conditions, including metabolic syndrome, growth abnormalities, and reproductive, immune, behavioral, or cognitive dysfunction in the offspring throughout their lifetime and even across subsequent generations.

The concept of developmental programming was first articulated by Dr David Barker and colleagues,[1,2] who used epidemiologic evidence in humans to show a strong association between low birth weight, poor postnatal environment, or other developmental insults, such as exposure to stress-related hormones (eg, corticoids), and the subsequent risk of developing, as adolescents and adults, the range of pathologic conditions noted above. Many subsequent epidemiologic studies in humans, as well as carefully controlled studies in other species, have confirmed these initial observations, and many of the risk factors for developmental programming have been identified (**Box 1**).[2,4–32]

Of relevance to this review article are the potential consequences for food animal production. In particular, many carefully controlled studies have shown that virtually every organ system and metabolic function are affected by developmental programming in livestock and other food animals (**Table 1**).

These observations beg the question, "Does developmental programming affect health and productivity of offspring in livestock?" Maternal nutritional status is a major factor in developmental programming events and ultimately offspring

---

Box 1
Risk factors for low birth weight/developmental programming

Risk factor

Lifestyle choices (humans only)
  Smoking, primarily associated with preterm birth
  Alcohol consumption, low birth weight/developmental disorders

Maternal factors (humans and/or animals)
  Poverty/lack of education/malnutrition
  Maternal age
  Ethnicity/breed/strain (genetic background)
  Maternal undernutrition or overnutrition
  Preterm birth and glucocorticoids
  Poor maternal health and/or health care status
  Sedentary lifestyle
  Maternal stress (eg, relational, social)
  Marital status

Environmental exposures (humans and animals)
  Herbicides, pesticides, and fungicides
  Other environmental exposures, for example, human waste/fertilizer, smoke, phytosteroids, drugs, temperature and humidity, high altitude

Adapted from Reynolds LP, Ward AK, Caton JS. Epigenetics and developmental programming in ruminants—long-term impacts on growth and development. In: Scanes CG, Hill R, editors. Biology of domestic animals. Milton Park (United Kingdom): CRC Press/Taylor & Francis Group; 2017. p. 85–121.

Table 1
Systems and bodily processes affected in the fetus and/or offspring during late pregnancy or postnatally in several models of developmental programming in livestock

Model	Systems and Processes Affected in the Fetus/Offspring During Late Pregnancy or Postnatally	Authors
Overfed adolescent or obese adult	Growth, body composition, energy balance, adipose, endocrine, gastrointestinal, muscle, reproductive	Abbot DH, Bartol FF, Alexander BT, Anthony RV, Bloomfield FH, Caton JS,
Underfed adolescent or adult	Brain, cardiovascular, endocrine, gastrointestinal, muscle, kidney, reproductive	Cunningham CP, Du M, Ford SP, Foxcroft G, Funston RN, Glover V,
Specific nutrients (eg, dietary protein or Se)	Growth, body composition, endocrine, gastrointestinal, reproductive	Greenwood P, McMillen IC, Nathanielsz PW, Padmanabhan V,
Multiple pregnancy	Behavior, endocrine, reproductive	Poston L, Reynolds LP,
Adolescent vs adult	Endocrine, reproductive	Robinson J, Symonds ME,
Maternal genotype (adult only)	Growth, gastrointestinal, reproductive	Vonnahme KA, Wallace JM, Wintour EM,
Behaviorally or environmentally stressed adult (including prenatal steroid exposure)	Behavior, growth, cardiovascular, endocrine, immune, reproductive	Wu G

This table is not comprehensive but rather lists results from some of the well-documented models of developmental programming in livestock. The authors' names are in a format that can be searched in PubMed (https://www.ncbi.nlm.nih.gov/pubmed/).

Adapted from Reynolds LP, Borowica PP, Caton JS, et al. Developmental programming: the concept, large animal models, and the key role of uteroplacental vascular development. J Anim Sci 2010;88(13):E61–72; with permission.

outcomes.[6,8,9,13,33] Prenatal growth trajectory is responsive to maternal nutrient intake from the early stages of embryonic life, when nutrient requirements for conceptus growth are reported to be negligible.[34–37] In ruminant livestock, because of seasonal changes in forage quality, and traditional approaches to supplementation, maternal nutrient restriction is usually thought of as the most likely nutritional issue facing producing female livestock.[13] However, during periods of confinement or lush forage growth, overconsumption and nutritional excess can be an issue, and data clearly show developmental programming of the offspring in response to excess maternal nutrition.[12,13] In addition to general nutrient restriction or excess, specific nutrient imbalances in the maternal diet can also have negative consequences for the developing offspring.[2,4–32] Because of the pattern of placental growth in relation to fetal growth during gestation, it also is important to realize that the effects of maternal nutrition during pregnancy may depend on the timing, level, or length of altered maternal diet.[13]

Although the concept of developmental programming was based on epidemiologic studies in humans, there was a hint of developmental programming, sometimes referred to as the maternal effect, for growth and productivity in livestock. For example, the classic crossbreeding experiment of Walton and Hammond[38,39] with large (Shire) and small (Shetland) horses showed that the uterine environment affects not only birth weight but also adult size (**Fig. 1**).

Unfortunately, there are few large data sets relating birth or weaning weights to long-term health and productivity in livestock. Recently, using a data set from the US Sheep Experiment Station for birth and weaning weights of more than 82,000

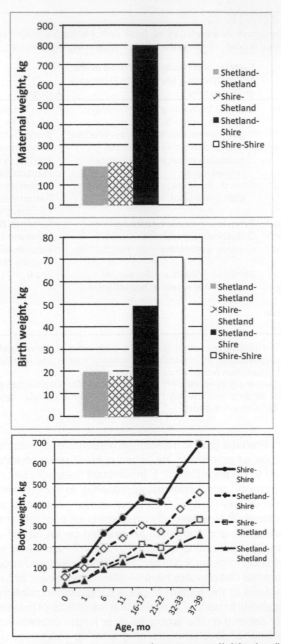

Fig. 1. Results of a crossbreeding experiment between small (Shetland) and large (Shire) horses. First breed indicates sire and second breed indicates dam. (*From* Reynolds LP, Ward AK, Caton JS. Epigenetics and developmental programming in ruminants—long-term impacts on growth and development. In: Scanes CG, Hill R, editors. Biology of domestic animals. Milton Park (United Kingdom): CRC Press/Taylor & Francis Group; 2017. p. 85–121; with permission.)

offspring across 5 decades, the authors found highly significant correlations between birth weight, weaning weight, and average daily gain to weaning.[13] Using the same data set, they also found highly significant effects of maternal age (yearling vs older dams) and fetal number (triplets vs singletons and twins) on mortality of the offspring due to pneumonia.[40] Similarly, using records from several thousand Nellore beef cattle, Chud and colleagues[41] recently reported a genetic correlation of 0.36 between birth weight and weaning weight and 0.20 between birth weight and accumulated productivity, which they defined as an index of dam efficiency that includes body weight of the calf at weaning (a growth trait) and number of offspring of the dam (a reproductive trait).

These recent observations using large data sets provide strong support for the idea that the profound effects of developmental programming that have been reported in carefully controlled studies with relatively small numbers of animals (see **Table 1**) do indeed, at least in some cases, result in increased morbidity and mortality, poor growth, and reduced productivity of offspring in livestock. In addition, although developmental programming is likely to negatively impact offspring productivity, perhaps the greatest consequence for livestock production is that the phenotype may not reflect the offspring's genetic potential, thereby leading to poorly informed selection decisions for breeding programs.[7,8]

An important point, however, is that developmental programming is not always bad. As the authors discuss briefly in later discussion, developmental programming and the resultant changes in organ structure, function, and gene expression serve to enable the developing fetus to adapt to environmental selection pressures relatively rapidly, much more so than evolution via genetic mutation (ie, natural selection). Thus, perturbations during fetal development, such as reduced maternal nutrient availability, can induce developmental changes that promote an energetically "thrifty" phenotype, leading to offspring that are better adapted to a nutrient-restricted environment postnatally.[42–44]

THE BASIS OF DEVELOPMENTAL PROGRAMMING
Placental Programming

After implantation, the placenta becomes the sole organ of exchange between the fetal and maternal systems. In other words, the fetus receives all of the nutrients and oxygen needed to support its development and also gives up its metabolic wastes to the mother solely via the placenta.[9,45–48] Because it is primarily an organ of transport, the placenta also develops an extensive blood supply (ie, it is highly vascular), which causes gravid uterine and umbilical blood flows (that represent the blood supplies to the maternal and fetal sides of the placenta, respectively) to increase exponentially throughout pregnancy, keeping pace with the exponential growth of the fetus.[9]

Many studies in livestock have shown that placental development and function are altered late in pregnancy in a variety of models of developmental programming, including maternal dietary intake (overfed or underfed), environmental heat stress, multiple pregnancy (singletons vs twins or triplets), adolescent versus adult pregnancies, and maternal breed (**Table 2**).

These observations agree with those in other species, including humans.[10,46,47] In addition, defects in placental growth, including vascular defects, normally precede altered fetal growth and development.[13,27,28] Importantly, the authors have shown that placental vascular development is affected during early gestation in compromised pregnancies.[49–54] Taken together, these observations have led to the concept of placental programming, that is, that altered placental growth and development are

Table 2
Reduced placental (uterine and umbilical) vascular development and blood flows in several models of compromised pregnancy in livestock[a]

Model	Fetal Weight, %	Placental Weight, %	Placental Vascular Development, %	Maternal Placental Blood Flow,[b] %	Fetal Placental Blood Flow,[b] %
Sheep					
Overfed adolescent	−30	−30	−31	−36	−37
Underfed adolescent	−17	NSE	−20	ND	ND
Underfed adult	−12	ND	−14	−25	NSE
Heat-stressed adult	−42	−51	ND	−26	−60
Multiple pregnancy[c]	−30	−37	−30	−23	ND
Adolescent vs adult[c]	−16	−26	−24	ND	ND
Maternal breed[c]	−44	−28	−33	ND	ND

ND, not determined; NSE, no significant effect.
[a] Reduced compared with noncompromised pregnancy; that is, pregnancy with normal fetal and placental size. All observations are from late pregnancy (day 130–135, approximately 0.9 of gestation).
[b] Maternal placental blood flow = blood flow to the pregnant uterus; fetal placental blood flow = umbilical blood flow.
[c] Multiple pregnancy compared singletons with triplets; adolescent versus adult were first pregnancies in the first season postnatally versus the second season postnatally; maternal breed compared Columbia with Romanov ewes.
Adapted from Reynolds LP, Caton JS, Redmer DA, et al. Evidence for altered placental blood flow and vascularity in compromised pregnancies. Invited (topical) review. J Physiol 2006;572(Pt 1):51–8; with permission.

important defects that underpin the altered fetal growth and organ development associated with developmental programming.[10,50]

Altered Growth and Development of Fetal Organs

In addition to placental programming, altered growth and development of fetal organs and organ systems can lead to (1) irreversible alterations in tissue and organ structure and organ size (ie, a structural defect), and (2) permanent changes in tissue function (ie, a permanent change in gene expression leading to a functional defect). Of course, in reality, structural and functional defects are intimately related, and their separate effects are difficult to resolve.

Structural defects that have been documented include changes in brown adipose deposition, altered nephron number leading to renal dysfunction, and altered pancreatic β-cell mass.[55–58] However, developmental programming of a structural defect is perhaps best exemplified by muscle, because the number of individual muscle cells (myocytes), or muscle fibers, is established before birth; after that, muscle fiber size can increase by the addition of nuclei from muscle satellite cells and subsequent hypertrophy, but no new muscle fibers can be added.[59,60] Muscle growth is therefore limited by the number of myocytes at birth. Thus, factors affecting fetal muscle development can lead to permanent, irreversible changes in muscle structure and growth potential.[60]

Muscle fiber number in offspring is affected by maternal nutrient restriction during pregnancy, and it has been argued that developing muscle is especially vulnerable to nutrient availability because of its low priority in terms of nutrient partitioning during fetal development, due primarily to its lower metabolic demands compared with tissues, such as brain, gut, and placenta, a concept first articulated by Sir Joseph Barcroft.[13,59,61] Maternal nutrient restriction, or other factors that limit nutrient availability, such as multiple fetuses, also affects development of other muscle cell types in addition to myocytes, including intramuscular adipocytes (which regulate intramuscular fat, or marbling) and fibroblasts (connective tissue-producing cells), leading to alterations in not only muscle size but also muscle marbling and connective tissue content in the offspring.[60]

As with most other organ systems, the period of pregnancy during which nutrient restriction is experienced determines which of these muscle cell types (ie, myocytes, adipocytes, or fibroblasts) is most affected.[60] That is, because it is the period of primary and secondary muscle fiber formation, maternal nutrient restriction during midgestation affects myocyte numbers and muscle mass in the offspring.[59] Conversely, because it is the period of skeletal muscle maturation, maternal nutrient restriction during late gestation does not affect myocyte numbers, but rather reduces myocyte size and affects the formation of intramuscular adipocytes.[59]

Altered Gene Expression due to Epigenetic Programming

Functional defects due to altered gene expression are best explained by a relatively novel concept termed "epigenetics," which literally translates to "above genetics," or "in addition to genetics," and is defined as heritable changes in gene expression without alteration of the genetic code. Epigenetic alterations are heritable through mitosis within an individual as well as transgenerationally through the germ line during reproduction.[9,10]

Epigenetic changes and the resultant changes in gene expression serve as a more rapid response in adaptation to environmental selection pressures than evolution via genetic mutation (ie, natural selection). Perturbations during fetal development, such as reduced nutrient availability, can induce epigenetic changes that promote an energetically "thrifty" phenotype, which, when exposed to a nutrient-rich environment, has increased risk of developing metabolic disease.[42–44] These alterations can persist through multiple generations, as exemplified by the pioneering studies by Ravelli and colleagues[62] of children born during the Dutch Famine (also called the Dutch Hunger Winter) of 1944 to 1945. Reduced intrauterine growth due to caloric restriction during gestation was associated with significant increases in type 2 diabetes and glucose intolerance in the offspring as adults.

Epigenetic mechanisms involve primarily 2 processes, methylation of DNA at cytosines in cytosine-guanosine (CpG) pairs and various modifications (methylation, acetylation, and so forth) of histones, which are the proteins around which DNA is wrapped. All of these processes determine whether a particular gene is "condensed" (also known as heterochromatin) and unavailable for transcription or, conversely, "open" (euchromatin) and ready to be transcribed (**Fig. 2**).[8,13] These epigenetic processes are not only altered by environmental factors but also heritable.[63,64]

Environmental factors that affect the epigenome, and thereby potentially have long-term and even transgenerational effects on gene expression and tissue/organ function, include nutrition, various environmental toxicants (eg, cigarette smoke, plasticizers, pesticides, herbicides), and social interactions (eg, spousal abuse, maternal care), and similar.[63,64] Most relevant to this discussion, when a pregnant woman or animal is subjected to these various environmental factors during pregnancy, the epigenome of her offspring is affected.[64]

As discussed, conditions during embryonic and fetal development, such as nutrient availability, shape the potential for growth and development through

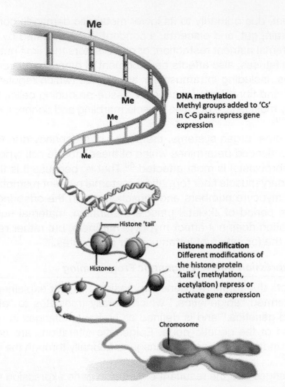

Fig. 2. The 2 main components of the "epigenetic code." (*From* Reynolds LP, Caton JS. Role of the pre- and post-natal environment in developmental programming of health and productivity. Mol Cell Endocrinol 2012;354:54–9; with permission.)

developmental programming. Epigenetic modification is probably a primary mechanism through which developmental programming effects are executed. Factors, such as maternal obesity, overnutrition, and nutrient deprivation, alter the trajectory of embryonic and fetal development, creating lasting effects that persist through to adulthood.

Maternal obesity is associated with metabolic dysregulation in the offspring, including insulin intolerance, obesity, and type 2 diabetes.[65,66] Studies in mice and rats have implicated epigenetic remodeling as the mechanism through which adipocyte differentiation is altered, ultimately leading to metabolic dysfunction later in development.[67,68] These studies found that maternal obesity altered the expression of genes regulating the development of adipocytes from precursor cells. Reduced promoter DNA methylation as well as histone methylation resulted in greater expression of the proadipogenic transcription factor Zfp423, leading to altered adipocyte differentiation within fetal tissues.

In cattle, maternal overnutrition during gestation is associated with increased fetal expression of markers of intramuscular adipogenesis. Fetuses collected at mid to late gestation from cows fed 150% of the maintenance requirements displayed increased expression of Zfp423, C/EBPα, and PPARγ, all of which are transcription factors involved in intramuscular adipocyte differentiation and proliferation.[69] Feeding a high-starch diet (vs a low-starch isocaloric and isonitrogenous control) from mid to late gestation resulted in calves with increased skeletal muscle expression of the DNA methyltransferase 3a as well the imprinted genes H19,

IGF2F, and MEG8, implying that maternal energy source alters epigenetic modulation.[70]

Maternal nutrient restriction is also associated with epigenetic changes that result in developmental programming. Rats that were feed-restricted by 50% during gestation produced pups with lower birth weight that displayed rapid compensatory growth and developed obesity and metabolic syndrome as adults.[71] Continuation of maternal feed restriction through lactation delayed the compensatory gain and prevented the development of obesity and metabolic syndrome in the offspring at maturity. The obese, gestationally feed-restricted rat pups reared by ad libitum–fed dams had significantly greater hepatic histone methylation of exon 1 and 2 of the IGF1 gene, and subsequently greater IGF1 expression than the nonobese, feed-restricted reared and control rats.

Protein restriction during pregnancy has been associated with epigenetically mediated dysregulation of glucocorticoid metabolism. In rats, protein restriction during gestation and lactation resulted in hypomethylation and increased expression of the hepatic glucocorticoid receptors.[72] Expression of methyl CpG-binding protein and its binding to the promoter of the glucocorticoid receptor gene was reduced, and multiple histone modifications were increased, implicating epigenetic alterations as the mechanism responsible for glucocorticoid dysregulation in the offspring.

EFFECTS OF MATERNAL STRESSORS DURING EARLY PREGNANCY ON FETAL GROWTH AND DEVELOPMENT

Early pregnancy is a critical period because of the major developmental events that take place, including embryonic organogenesis as well as formation of the placenta, a process known as placentation.[54,73,74] The authors recently evaluated the pattern of placental vascular growth and development during early pregnancy after natural breeding in sheep and demonstrated that the major initial changes appear in the endometrium (the maternal portion of the placenta) very early in pregnancy (as early as day 16 after mating).[54,73,74] In addition, changes in vascularization measured by area, surface, number, and density of capillaries were highly correlated with changes in expression of several angiogenic factors in maternal placenta.[54,73,74] For several other species (eg, humans, marmoset, rats), intensive vascular development in placenta was also observed during first 3 to 4 weeks of pregnancy and was associated with enhanced metabolic demand to support dramatic fetal growth.[54,73,74]

Comparison of placental development in natural pregnancies and pregnancies achieved by various assisted reproductive techniques (ART), such as after transfer of embryos created through cloning or in vitro fertilization (IVF), has demonstrated numerous significant effects of ART on placental and fetal growth and development as well as offspring outcome in several species.[54,73,74] In various animals, including mice, cattle, and sheep, impaired placental steroid metabolism, abnormal offspring syndrome, increased duration of gestation, altered placental vascularization, and altered fetal weight or size, and placenta:fetus ratio have been reported after using ART.[54,73,74] For early pregnancy in cows, both greater and lesser crown-rump length have been reported for fetuses created in vitro and then transferred compared with fetuses created in vivo.[75,76]

In sheep, the authors and others have recently demonstrated that utero-placental vascularization, expression of several angiogenic factors, receptors for P4 and estrogens, and DNA methyl transferases, as well as global DNA methylation and markers of growth, all were altered in the developing placenta during early pregnancy after transfer of embryos obtained through IVF or in vitro activation (parthenotes, which have only a maternal genome).[54,73,74] These observations suggest that changes in DNA methylation or histone modifications observed in early embryos of several species (cattle, mice, sheep) after ART[77–81] continue during the critical period of placentation during early pregnancy. In addition, based on observations later in pregnancy, the authors have suggested that these placental developmental defects probably contribute to poor placental vascularization and function later in pregnancy, ultimately leading to altered fetal growth/development and poor pregnancy outcomes associated with ART.[54,73,74] Such epigenetic defects leading to altered placental gene expression and development have been observed after IVF and especially in clones not only in sheep but also in cattle and mice.[82] These defects include altered expression of imprinted genes, which are thought to be critical for normal placental development.[83–85]

In the last several years, the authors have begun looking at the effects of maternal nutrient restriction during the first 50 days of pregnancy on fetoplacental development in beef heifers, using a standing, flank ovariohysterectomy procedure that they developed.[86] Using this model, they found altered expression of endogenous retroviruses and interferon-tau, both of which are important in placentation and establishment of pregnancy, in the developing placental tissues of nutrient-restricted compared with control-fed heifers as early as day 16 after mating.[87] In addition, the authors found that nutrient-restricted heifers had altered placental expression of angiogenic factors and associated alterations in placental vascular development.[53]

Using this same model, pregnant heifers that were nutrient restricted during early pregnancy also exhibited dramatically altered gene expression in fetal organs. Using RNAseq, the authors evaluated gene expression in fetal liver, muscle, and brain (cerebrum) on day 50 after mating.[88] They found that 201, 144, and 28 genes were differentially expressed in fetal liver, muscle, and brain, respectively, in nutrient-restricted compared with control-fed heifers. In addition, many of the differentially expressed genes were relatively tissue specific; for example, genes involved in metabolic pathways and complement-coagulation cascades in liver, skeletal muscle-specific genes in muscle, and hippocampus- and neurogenesis-related genes in brain.[88]

These observations suggest that 50 days of very moderate nutrient restriction during early pregnancy, which could be expected to occur under extensive management systems in beef heifers or in ewes, especially on native range, not only profoundly affects gene expression in the fetal organs and placenta but also may set up the pregnancy for failure or, perhaps more likely, alter fetal and placental development and, ultimately, developmental programming of postnatal health and productivity. Thus, despite the fact that fetal and placental growth are minimal during the first 50 days of pregnancy, the many critical events that take place, including fetal organogenesis and placentation, appear to be susceptible to poor maternal nutrition.

An important point, however, is that despite the dramatic effects of maternal undernutrition on fetal organs, fetal size was not affected by maternal undernutrition during early pregnancy in beef heifers (**Fig. 3**). Thus, just as for placental vascular development, altered gene expression precedes any detectable effects on organ, or in this case, fetal size.[10,48,53,75,87,89,90] Another important point is that not only does maternal nutrition during early pregnancy affect embryonic/fetal development but also even premating nutritional plane, and by extension body condition at mating, has dramatic effects on embryonic development and developmental outcomes. For example, in sheep, underfeeding or overfeeding for 8 weeks before oocyte collection dramatically reduces the rates of IVF and subsequent embryonic development.[91] Similarly, underfeeding of ewes for 60 days before until 30 days after mating resulted in early delivery

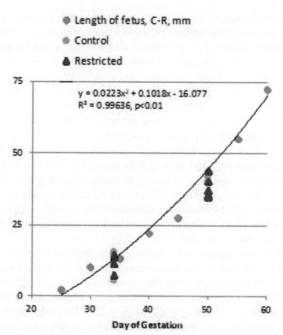

Fig. 3. Fetal size (crown-rump length, CR, in millimeters) in beef heifers from size day 16 to 60 of pregnancy; control-fed (green circles) versus restricted-fed (red triangles) heifers were evaluated only on days 34 and 50. (*Data from* Pereira NN, Dahlen CR, Borowicz PP, et al. Fetal and placental growth during the first 90 days of gestation in beef heifers, and effects of maternal nutrition. J Anim Sci 2017;95(suppl 4):150–1.)

(6–11 days early compared with control-fed ewes) of dysmature lambs, all of whom died soon after birth.[92–94]

STRATEGIES TO MINIMIZE THE EFFECTS OF DEVELOPMENTAL PROGRAMMING

The most obvious way to minimize the negative consequences of developmental programming is to simply ensure that maternal nutrition is optimal, and this approach has a great deal of merit. For example, the authors have shown that the level of metabolizable protein in the maternal diet affects birth weights of the offspring in both cattle and sheep.[95,96] Other researchers have also shown that beef cattle grazing dormant range but receiving protein supplementation during the last one-third of pregnancy produce heifer calves with reduced age at puberty and increased first pregnancy rate compared with heifer calves from nonsupplemented dams.[97,98] However, Tanner and coworkers[99] reported no effects of corn supplementation during the last two-thirds of pregnancy on calf size at birth in multiparous cows receiving a low-quality, forage-based total mixed ration. Thus, the effects of supplementation may depend on the quality of the diet in the nonsupplemented controls, on the specific nutrients supplied, or on the timing of supplementation.

Another approach to minimize the effects of developmental programming is to use dietary supplementation that targets specific processes. For example, the authors have shown in sheep that maternal dietary selenium supplementation at "supernutritional" but subtoxic levels may protect fetal or neonatal organ systems from the negative effects of dietary restriction during pregnancy.[100,101] Another example involves several amino acids, including many of the essential amino acids, which have been termed functional amino acids because they not only serve as building blocks of proteins but also regulate, directly or indirectly, key metabolic pathways necessary for growth, reproduction, immunity, and so forth.[102] The amino acid arginine (Arg) is the immediate precursor for at least 2 critical processes, as follows: (1) the production of nitric oxide, which is an important vasodilator (ie, it causes blood vessels to dilate and thus enhances cardiovascular function); and (2) the production of polyamines, which are critical for normal cell and tissue growth.[102] It has been shown that dietary supplementation of gilts with Arg during pregnancy increases the number of piglets born alive and live litter birth weights.[103] In addition, Lassala and coworkers[104] showed that intravenous infusion of Arg 3 times daily from day 60 until parturition was able to rescue birth weights of lambs in ewes receiving only 50% of National Research Council nutrient requirements from day 28 of pregnancy onwards. Similarly, the authors have shown that intravenous administration of Arg once daily from the day of mating through day 15 of gestation increases embryo survival and decreases embryo loss in ewes of low prolificacy.[105]

Other essential amino acids and vitamins, including methionine, serine, glycine, choline, vitamin B_{12}, and folate, are involved in DNA and histone methylation, or 1-carbon metabolism. It has been shown that dietary levels of these amino acids and vitamins can dramatically affect epigenetic regulation of gene expression and can reduce the incidence of diseases or developmental defects.[63,64] Whether these dietary factors can minimize the epigenetic-dependent negative consequences of developmental programming remains to be determined. However, in a recent study in which a rumen-protected formulation of methionine was fed during the last 28 days of pregnancy in dairy cows, calves were larger at birth compared with those born to cows not receiving methionine supplementation, and these calves also exhibited greater average daily gain and body weight through 9 weeks of age.[106] This observation agrees with reports that dietary supplementation with methyl donors (methionine as well as choline, betaine, folate, and vitamin B_{12}) in pregnant mice reduces the incidence of obesity, metabolic syndrome, altered feeding behavior, and cancer susceptibility in the offspring.[107–110]

Additional therapeutic/management approaches are those designed to directly impact placental blood flow using pharmacologic agents. For example, Satterfield and colleagues[111] administered sildenafil, which is marketed under the trade name Viagra, from day 28 until day 115 in pregnant, nutrient-restricted ewes and found that fetal weights were similar to those of control-fed ewes and greater than those of nutrient-restricted ewes not receiving sildenafil. Interestingly, in that study fetal weight also was greater in control-fed ewes receiving sildenafil compared with those not receiving sildenafil.

Another approach has been to supplement with melatonin, which has been shown to affect oxidative status, steroid and prostaglandin metabolism, and cardiovascular function.[112] In these studies, melatonin supplementation during the last two-thirds of pregnancy was able to improve umbilical blood flow and fetal growth in melatonin compared with non-melatonin-fed ewes, whether or not they were fed a control or a restricted diet.[112] Similarly, melatonin supplementation of pregnant beef heifers during the last half of pregnancy resulted in increased uterine artery blood flow and increased body weight and scrotal circumference of the male offspring at weaning.[113]

SUMMARY

Although the large data sets combining birth and placental weights, maternal and postnatal nutrition, and health records are sparse for food animals, many controlled studies have demonstrated that developmental insults lead to altered growth, metabolism, and reproductive, immune, behavioral, and cognitive dysfunction in livestock. The few large data sets that have been evaluated suggest that, just as in humans, developmental insults associated with compromised fetal and postnatal growth and development have long-term consequences, ultimately affecting the productivity of the offspring. An additional and poorly recognized consequence of developmental programming is that it will affect the phenotype of the offspring, such that the phenotype will not reflect the offspring's genetic potential, thereby leading to poorly informed selection decisions for breeding programs.

The good news is that many of the risk factors for low birth weight/developmental programming have been identified, as have many of the mechanisms that are responsible for the long-term programming or organ/system structure and function. Thus, numerous strategies, including improved diet, targeted dietary supplementation, and therapeutics designed to improve gene expression of and nutrient delivery to the fetus, are being examined. These and other strategies must continue to be investigated because they hold promise for not only "rescuing" fetal growth and development but also reducing the negative consequences of developmental programming in livestock. Conversely, research focused on the potential positive, adaptive, benefits of developmental programming is sorely needed.

It will be up to animal scientists and veterinarians to ensure that farmers, ranchers, policy makers, and the public in general recognize the factors causing developmental programming as well as the potential consequences, whether dire or beneficial. It also will be critical that they recognize the importance of continued research in this area.

ACKNOWLEDGMENTS

Our research over the last thirty years has been supported primarily by the U.S. National Institute of Food and Agriculture, National Institutes of Health, and National Science Foundation, as well as the North Dakota Agricultural Experiment Station and the North Dakota State Board of Agricultural Research and Education.

REFERENCES

1. Barker DJP. Fetal and infant origins of adult disease. London: BMJ Publishing Group; 1992.
2. Barker DJP. Developmental origins of well being. Philos Trans R Soc Lond B Biol Sci 2004;359:1359–66.
3. Paneth N, Susser M. Early origin of coronary heart disease (the "Barker hypothesis"). Br Med J 1995;1310:411–2.
4. Armitage JA, Khan IY, Taylor PD, et al. Developmental programming of the metabolic syndrome by maternal nutritional imbalance: how strong is the evidence from experimental models in mammals? J Physiol 2004;561:355–77.
5. Wu G, Bazer FW, Wallace JM, et al. Intrauterine growth retardation: implications for the animal sciences. J Anim Sci 2006;84:2316–37.
6. Caton JS, Hess BW. Maternal plane of nutrition: impacts on fetal outcomes and postnatal offspring responses [Invited Review]. In: Hess BW, Delcurto T, Bowman JGP, et al, editors. Proc. 4th grazing livestock nutrition conference. 2010. p. 104–22. Proc. West Sect. Am. Soc. Anim. Sci., Champaign (IL).
7. Reynolds LP, Borowica PP, Caton JS, et al. Developmental programming: the concept, large animal models, and the key role of uteroplacental vascular development. J Anim Sci 2010b;88(13):E61–72.

8. Reynolds LP, Caton JS. Role of the pre- and post-natal environment in developmental programming of health and productivity. Mol Cell Endocrinol 2012;354: 54–9.

9. Reynolds LP, Borowicz PP, Caton JS, et al. Uteroplacental vascular development and placental function: an update. Int J Dev Biol 2010a;54(2–3):355–66.

10. Reynolds LP, Vonnahme KA. Livestock as models for developmental programming [Invited Review]. Animal Frontiers 2017;7:12–7.

11. Luther JS, Redmer DA, Reynolds LP, et al. Nutritional paradigms of ovine fetal growth restriction: implications for human pregnancy. Hum Fertil 2005;8:179–87.

12. Wallace JM, Luther JS, Milne JS, et al. Nutritional modulation of adolescent pregnancy outcome–a review. Placenta 2006;27(a):S61–8.

13. Reynolds LP, Ward AK, Caton JS. Epigenetics and developmental programming in ruminants–long-term impacts on growth and development. In: Scanes CG, Hill R, editors. Biology of domestic animals. Milton Park (United Kingdom): CRC Press/Taylor & Francis Group; 2017. p. 85–121.

14. Aizer A, Currie J. The intergenerational transmission of inequality: maternal disadvantage and health at birth. Science 2014;344:856–61.

15. Alfaradhi MZ, Ozanne SE. Developmental programming in response to maternal overnutrition. Front Genet 2011;2:1–13.

16. Armitage JA, Taylor PD, Poston L. Experimental models of developmental programming: consequences of exposure to an energy rich diet during development. J Physiol 2005;565(Pt 1):3–8.

17. Been JV, Nurmatov UB, Cox B, et al. Effect of smoke-free legislation on perinatal and child health: a systematic review and meta-analysis. Lancet 2014;383: 1549–60.

18. Bellingham M, Fowler PA, Amezaga MR, et al. Foetal hypothalamic and pituitary expression of gonadotrophin-releasing hormone and galanin systems is disturbed by exposure to sewage sludge chemicals via maternal ingestion. J Neuroendocrinol 2010;22:527–33.

19. Brunton PJ. Effects of maternal exposure to social stress during pregnancy: consequences for mother and offspring. Reproduction 2013;146:R175–89.

20. Crain DA, Janssen SJ, Edwards TM, et al. Female reproductive disorders: the role of endocrine-disrupting compounds and developmental timing. Fertil Steril 2008;90:911–40.

21. Dupont C, Cordier AG, Junien C, et al. Maternal environment and reproductive function of the offspring. Theriogenology 2012;78:1405–14.

22. Evans NP, Bellingham M, Sharpe RM, et al. Reproduction Symposium: does grazing on biosolids-treated pasture pose a pathophysiological risk associated with increased exposure to endocrine disrupting compounds? J Anim Sci 2014; 92:3185–98.

23. Fowden AL, Forhead AJ. Hormones as epigenetic signals in developmental programming. Exp Physiol 2009;94(6):607–25.

24. Fowden AL, Giussani DA, Forhead AJ. Intrauterine programming of physiological systems: causes and consequences. Physiology (Bethesda) 2006;21: 29–37.

25. Fowler PA, Bellingham M, Sinclair KD, et al. Impact of endocrine-disrupting compounds (EDCs) on female reproductive health. Mol Cell Endocrinol 2012; 355:231–9.

26. Galbally M, Snellen M, Power J. Antipsychotic drugs in pregnancy: a review of their maternal and fetal effects. Ther Adv Drug Saf 2014;52:100–9.

27. Harris EK, Berg EP, Berg EL, et al. Effect of maternal activity during gestation on maternal behavior, fetal growth, umbilical blood flow, and farrowing characteristics in pigs. J Anim Sci 2013;91:734–44.
28. Juul A, Almstrup K, Andersson A-M, et al. Possible fetal determinants of male infertility. Nat Rev Endocrinol 2014;10:553–62.
29. Li M, Sloboda DM, Vickers MH. Maternal obesity and developmental programming of metabolic disorders in offspring: evidence from animal models. Exp Diabetes Res 2011;2011:592408.
30. Schneider JE, Brozek JM, Keen-Rhinehart E. Our stolen figures: the interface of sexual differentiation, endocrine disruptors, maternal programming, and energy balance. Horm Behav 2014;66:110–9.
31. Seneviratne SN, Parry GK, McCowan LME, et al. Antenatal exercise in overweight and obese women and its effects on offspring and maternal health: design and rationale of the IMPROVE (Improving Maternal and Progeny Obesity Via Exercise) randomized controlled trial. BMC Pregnancy Childbirth 2014;14: 148. Available at: http://www.biomedcentral.com/1471-2393/14/148.
32. Skinner MK. Endocrine disruptor induction of epigenetic transgenerational inheritance of disease. Mol Cell Endocrinol 2014;398:4–12.
33. Funston R,N, Summers AF, Roberts AJ. Alpharma Beef Cattle Nutrition Symposium: implications of nutritional management for beef cow-calf systems. J Anim Sci 2012;90:2301–7.
34. Meyer AM, Caton JS. The role of the small intestine in developmental programming: impact of maternal nutrition on the dam and offspring. Adv Nutr 2016;7: 160 70.
35. Robinson JJ, Sinclair KD, McEvoy TG. Nutritional effects on foetal growth. Anim Sci 1999;68:315–31.
36. National Research Council (NRC). Nutrient requirements of beef cattle. 7th revised edition. Washington, DC: National Academy Press; 1996.
37. National Research Council (NRC). Nutrients requirements of small ruminants, sheep, goats, cervids and new world camelids. Washington, DC: The National Academies Press.; 2007.
38. Hammond J. The physiology of reproduction in the cow. Cambridge (United Kingdom): Cambridge University Press; 1927.
39. Walton A, Hammond J. The maternal effects on growth and conformation in Shire horse-Shetland pony crosses. Proceedings of the Royal Society B 1938; 125:311–35.
40. Holland PW, Hulsman Hanna LL, Vonnahme KA, et al. Genetic parameters for lamb mortality associated with pneumonia. J Anim Sci 2018;96(Suppl. 1):1. Proceedings Southern Section, American Society of Animal Sciences.
41. Chud TCS, Caetano SL, Buzankas ME, et al. Genetic analysis for gestation length, birth weight, weaning weight, and accumulated productivity in Nellore beef cattle. Livest Sci 2014;170:16–21.
42. Hales CN, Barker DJ. The thrifty phenotype hypothesis. Br Med Bull 2001;60: 5–20.
43. Wells JCK. The thrifty phenotype as an adaptive maternal effect. Biol Rev Camb Philos Soc 2007;82:13–72.
44. Vaag AA, Grunnet LG, Arora GP, et al. The thrifty phenotype hypothesis revisited. Diabetologia 2012;55:2085–8.
45. Reynolds LP, Caton JS, Redmer DA, et al. Evidence for altered placental blood flow and vascularity in compromised pregnancies [Invited (Topical) Review]. J Physiol 2006;572(Pt 1):51–8.

46. Mayhew TM, Wijesekara J, Baker PN, et al. Short communication: morphometric evidence that villous development and fetoplacental angiogenesis are compromised by intrauterine growth restriction but not by pre-eclampsia. Placenta 2004;25:829–33.

47. Mayhew TM. A stereological perspective on placental morphology in normal and complicated pregnancies. J Anat 2009;215:77–90.

48. Redmer DA, Aitken RP, Milne JS, et al. Influence of maternal nutrition on messenger RNA expression of placental angiogenic factors and their receptors at mid-gestation in adolescent sheep. Biol Reprod 2005;72:1004–9.

49. Vonnahme KA, Zhu MJ, Borowicz PP, et al. Effect of early gestational undernutrition on angiogenic factor expression and vascularity in the bovine placentome. J Anim Sci 2007;85:2464–72.

50. Vonnahme KA, Lemley CO, Shukla P, et al. Placental programming: how the maternal environment can impact placental function. J Anim Sci 2013;91:2467–80.

51. Grazul-Bilska AT, Johnson ML, Borowicz PP, et al. Placental development during early pregnancy in sheep: effects of embryo origin on fetal and placental growth and global methylation. Theriogenology 2013;79:94–102.

52. Grazul-Bilska AT, Johnson ML, Borowicz PP, et al. Placental development during early pregnancy in sheep: effects of embryo origin on vascularization. Reproduction 2014;147:639–48.

53. McLean KJ, Crouse MS, Crosswhite MR, et al. Impacts of maternal nutrition on placental vascularity and mRNA expression of angiogenic factors during the establishment of pregnancy in beef heifers. Transl Anim Sci 2017;1:160–7.

54. Bairagi S, Quinn KE, Crane AR, et al. Maternal environment and placental vascularization in domestic ruminants [Invited Review]. Theriogenology 2016;86:288–305.

55. Symonds ME, Pope M, Sharkey D, et al. Adipose tissue and fetal programming. Diabetologia 2012;55:1597–606.

56. Richter VFI, Briffa JF, Moritz KM, et al. The role of maternal nutrition, metabolic function and the placental in developmental programming of renal dysfunction. Clin Exp Pharmacol Physiol 2016;43:135–41.

57. Martin-Gronert MS, Ozanne SE. Metabolic programming of insulin action and secretion. Diabetes Obes Metab 2012;14(3):29–39.

58. Gatford KL, Simmons RA. Prenatal programming of insulin secretion in intrauterine growth restriction. Clin Obstet Gynecol 2013;56:520–8.

59. Du M, Tong J, Zhao J, et al. Fetal programming of skeletal muscle development in ruminant animals. J Anim Sci 2010;88:E51–60.

60. Du M, Zhao JX, Yan X, et al. Fetal muscle development, mesenchymal multipotent cell differentiation and associated signaling pathways. J Anim Sci 2011;89:583–90.

61. Barcroft J. Researches on pre-natal life. Oxford: Blackwell; 1946.

62. Ravelli ACJ, van der Meulen JHP, Michels RPJ, et al. Glucose tolerance in adults after prenatal exposure to famine. Lancet 1998;351:173–7.

63. Jaenisch R, Bird A. Epigenetic regulation of gene expression: how the genome integrates intrinsic and environmental signals. Nat Genet 2003;33(Suppl):245–54.

64. Skinner MK, Manikkam M, Guerrero-Bosagna C. Epigenetic transgenerational actions of environmental factors in disease etiology. Trends Endocrinol Metab 2010;21(4):214–22.

65. Shankar K, Harrell A, Liu X, et al. Maternal obesity at conception programs obesity in the offspring. Am J Physiol Regul Integr Comp Physiol 2008;294: R528–38.
66. Shankar K, Kang P, Harrell A, et al. Maternal overweight programs insulin and adiponectin signaling in the offspring. Endocrinology 2010;151:2577–89.
67. Yang QY, Liang JF, Rogers CJ, et al. Maternal obesity induces epigenetic modifications to facilitate Zfp423 expression and enhance adipogenic differentiation in fetal mice. Diabetes 2013;62:3727–35.
68. Borengasser SJ, Zhong Y, Kang P, et al. Maternal obesity enhances white adipose tissue differentiation and alters genome-scale DNA methylation in male rat offspring. Endocrinology 2013;154:4113–25.
69. Duarte MS, Gionbelli MP, Paulino PVR, et al. Maternal overnutrition enhances mRNA expression of adipogenic markers and collagen deposition in skeletal muscle of beef cattle fetuses. J Anim Sci 2014;92:3846–54.
70. Wang X, Lan X, Radunz AE, et al. Maternal nutrition during pregnancy is associated with differential expression of imprinted genes and DNA methyltransferases in muscle of beef cattle offspring. J Anim Sci 2015;93:35–40.
71. Tosh DN, Fu Q, Callaway CW, et al. Epigenetics of programmed obesity: alteration of IUGR rat hepatic IGF1 mRNA expression and histone structure in rapid vs. delayed postnatal catch-up growth. Am J Physiol Gastrointest Liver Physiol 2010;299:G1023–9.
72. Lillycrop KA, Slater-Jefferies JL, Hanson MA, et al. Induction of altered epigenetic regulation of the hepatic glucocorticoid receptor in the offspring of rats fed a protein-restricted diet during pregnancy suggests that reduced DNA methyltransferase-1 expression is involved in impaired DNA methylation and changes in histone modification. Br J Nutr 2007;97:1064–73.
73. Reynolds LP, Vonnahme KA, Lemley CO, et al. Maternal stress and placental vascular function and remodeling. Curr Vasc Pharmacol 2013;11:564–93.
74. Reynolds LP, Borowicz PP, Palmieri C, et al. Placental vascular defects in compromised pregnancies: effects of assisted reproductive technologies and other maternal stressors. In: Zhang L, Ducsay CA, editors. Advances in fetal and neonatal physiology. Advances in Experimental Medicine and Biology, vol. 814. New York: Springer Science+Business Media; 2014. p. 193–204.
75. Bertolini M, Mason JB, Beam SW, et al. Morphology and morphometry of in vivo- and in vitro-produced bovine concepti from early pregnancy to term and association with high birth weights. Theriogenology 2002;58(5):973–94.
76. Farin PW, Piedrahita JA, Farin CE. Errors in development of fetuses and placentas from in vitro-produced bovine embryos. Theriogenology 2006;65: 178–91.
77. Bourc'his D, Le Bourhis D, Patin D, et al. Delayed and incomplete reprogramming of chromosome methylation patterns in bovine cloned embryos. Curr Biol 2001;11:1542–6.
78. Beaujean N, Taylor J, Gardner J, et al. Effect of limited DNA methylation reprogramming in the normal sheep embryo on somatic cell nuclear transfer. Biol Reprod 2004;71:185–93.
79. Suteevun T, Parnpai R, Smith SL, et al. Epigenetic characteristics of cloned and in vitro-fertilized swamp buffalo (Bubalus bubalis) embryos. J Anim Sci 2006;84: 2065–71.
80. de Waal E, Yamazaki Y, Ingale P, et al. Gonadotropin stimulation contributes to an increased incidence of epimutations in ICSI-derived mice. Hum Mol Genet 2012;21:4460–72.

81. de Waal E, Yamazaki Y, Ingale P, et al. Primary epimutations introduced during intracytoplasmic sperm injection (ICSI) are corrected by germline-specific epigenetic reprogramming. Proc Natl Acad Sci U S A 2012;109:4163–8.
82. Palmieri C, Loi P, Ptak G, et al. Review paper: a review of the pathology of abnormal placentae of somatic cell nuclear transfer clone pregnancies in cattle, sheep, and mice. Vet Pathol 2008;45:865–80.
83. Bressan FF, De Bem THC, Perecin F, et al. Unearthing the roles of imprinted genes in the placenta. Placenta 2009;30:823–34.
84. Mesquita FS, Machado SA, Drnevich J, et al. Influence of cloning by chromatin transfer on placental gene expression at Day 45 of pregnancy in cattle. Anim Reprod Sci 2013;136:231–44.
85. Ptak GE, D'Agostino A, Toschi P, et al. Post-implantation mortality of in vitro produced embryos is associated with DNA methyltransferase I dysfunction in sheep placenta. Hum Reprod 2013;28:298–305.
86. McLean KJ, Dahlen CR, Borowicz PP, et al. Technical note: a new surgical technique for ovariohysterectomy during early pregnancy in beef heifers. J Anim Sci 2016;94:5089–96.
87. McLean KJ, Crouse MS, Crosswhite MR, et al. The effects of nutrient restriction on mRNA expression of endogenous retroviruses, interferon-tau, and pregnancy specific protein-B during the establishment of pregnancy in beef heifers. J Anim Sci 2018;96:950–63.
88. Crouse MS, Caton JS, Cushman RA, et al. Moderate nutrient restriction of beef heifers alters expression of genes associated with tissue metabolism, accretion, and function in fetal liver, muscle, and cerebrum by d 50 of gestation. Trans Anim Sci (In Press). doi: 10.1093/tas/txz026.
89. Redmer DA, Luther J, Milne J, et al. J. Fetoplacental growth and vascular development in overnourished adolescent sheep at day 50, 90 and 130 of gestation. Reproduction 2009;137:749–57.
90. Barnes FL. The effects of the early uterine environment on the subsequent development of embryo and fetus. Theriogenology 2000;53:649–58.
91. Grazul-Bilska AT, Borowczyk E, Bilski JJ, et al. Overfeeding and underfeeding have detrimental effects on oocyte quality measured by in vitro fertilization and early embryonic development in sheep. Domest Anim Endocrinol 2012; 43:289–98.
92. Bloomfield FH, Oliver MH, Hawkins P, et al. A periconceptional nutritional origin for noninfectious preterm birth. Science 2003;300:606.
93. Kumarasamy V, Mitchell MD, Bloomfield FH, et al. Effects of periconceptional undernutrition on the initiation of parturition in sheep. Am J Physiol Regul Integr Comp Physiol 2005;288:R67–72.
94. Oliver MH, Jaquiery AL, Bloomfield FH, et al. The effects of maternal nutrition around the time of conception on the health of the offspring. Soc Reprod Fertil Suppl 2007;64:397–410.
95. Sletmoen-Olson KE, Caton JS, Olson KC, et al. Undegraded intake protein supplementation: I. Effects on forage utilization and performance of periparturient beef cows fed low-quality hay. J Anim Sci 2000;78:449–55.
96. O'Rourke ST, Modgil A, Sun C, et al. Maternal dietary protein level alters function of large-conductance, calcium-activated k (bkca) channels in fetal coronary arterial smooth muscle cells. Pediatr Res 2010;68:177.
97. Funston RN, Larson DM, Vonnahme KA. Effects of maternal nutrition on conceptus growth and offspring performance: implications for beef cattle production. J Anim Sci 2010;88: E205–215E.

98. Broadhead D, Mulliniks JT, Funston RN. Developmental programming in a beef production system. Vet Clin Food Anim 2019;35(2):381–92.
99. Tanner AR, Kennedy VC, Bauer ML, et al. Corn supplementation as a winter-feeding strategy alters maternal feeding behavior and endocrine profiles in mid- to late-gestating beef cows. Transl Anim Sci 2018;2:S106–11.
100. Reed JJ, Ward MA, Vonnahme KA, et al. Effects of selenium supply and dietary restriction on maternal and fetal body weight, visceral organ mass, cellularity estimates, and jejunal vascularity in pregnant ewe lambs. J Anim Sci 2007;85: 2721–33.
101. Meyer AM, Reed JJ, Neville TL, et al. Effects of plane of nutrition and selenium supply during gestation on ewe and neonatal offspring performance, body composition, and serum selenium. J Anim Sci 2010;88(5):1786–800.
102. Wu G. Amino acids: metabolism, functions, and nutrition. Amino Acids 2009; 37(1):1–17.
103. Mateo RD, Wu G, Bazer FW, et al. Dietary L-arginine supplementation enhances the reproductive performance of gilts. J Nutr 2007;137(3):652–6.
104. Lassala A, Bazer FW, Cudd TA, et al. Parenteral administration of L-arginine prevents fetal growth restriction in undernourished ewes. J Nutr 2010;140(7): 1242–8.
105. Luther JS, Windorski EJ, Schauer CS, et al. Impacts of L-arginine on ovarian function and reproductive performance in ewes. J Anim Sci 2008;86(E-Suppl. 2):ii [abstract].
106. Alharthi AS, Batister F, Abdelmegeld MK, et al. Maternal supply of methionine during late pregnancy enhances rate of Holstein calf development in utero and postnatal growth to a greater extent than colostrum source. J Anim Sci Biotechnol 2018;9:83.
107. Dolinoy DC. The agouti mouse model: an epigenetic biosensor for nutritional and environmental alterations on the fetal epigenome. Nutr Rev 2008;66:S7–11.
108. Cooney CA, Dave AA, Wolff GL. Maternal methyl supplements in mice affect epigenetic variation and DNA methylation of offspring. J Nutr 2002;132: 2393S–400S.
109. Carlin J, George R, Reyes TM. Methyl donor supplementation blocks the adverse effects of maternal high fat diet on offspring physiology. PLoS One 2013;8:e63549.
110. Cho K, Mabasa L, Bae S, et al. Maternal high-methyl diet suppresses mammary carcinogenesis in female rat offspring. Carcinogenesis 2012;33:1106–12.
111. Satterfield MC, Bazer FW, Spencer TE, et al. Sildenafil citrate treatment enhances amino acid availability in the conceptus and fetal growth in an ovine model of intrauterine growth restriction. J Nutr 2010;140:251–8.
112. Lemley CO, Meyer AM, Camacho LE, et al. Melatonin supplementation alters uteroplacental hemodynamics and fetal development in an ovine model of intrauterine growth restriction. Am J Physiol Regul Integr Comp Physiol 2012;302: R454–67.
113. McCarty KJ, Owen MPT, Hart CG, et al. Effect of chronic melatonin supplementation during mid to late gestation on maternal uterine artery blood flow and subsequent development of male offspring in beef cattle. J Anim Sci 2018;96(12): 5100–11.

Cellular Mechanisms and Epigenetic Changes
Role of Nutrition in Livestock

Ahmed Elolimy, MS, Mario Vailati-Riboni, MS, Yusheng Liang, MS, Juan J. Loor, PhD*

KEYWORDS

- Embryo • Histones • Methylation • Placenta • Pregnancy • Tissue

KEY POINTS

- Epigenetic events occurring via DNA methylation, posttranslational modifications of histones, and abundance of microRNA are required for normal development of tissues at various stages of the life cycle.
- Maternal nutrition of livestock during pregnancy can alter the fetal and postnatal epigenome and transcriptome, often leading to measurable alterations in metabolism and growth.
- A shortfall in the total dietary supply of nutrients, vitamin B_{12}, folate, betaine, choline, or methionine during key stages of the life cycle can alter epigenetic mechanisms.
- Epigenomics and physiologic and developmental outcomes offer exciting opportunities for in-depth discoveries of potentially crucial modifications of DNA and histones that can impact efficiency of nutrient use and well-being of livestock.

INTRODUCTION

Ample evidence from research with humans and model organisms demonstrates the unique role that epigenetic mechanisms have on basic development, growth, physiology, and health. Epigenetic changes or marks not only are transmitted from cells to cells during cell division, but from mother to offspring and can be compiled into the epigenome. From an environmental standpoint, the recognition that nutrition can alter the profile of the epigenome even among individuals with identical genetic code has increased interest among livestock scientists for a better understanding of the implications of adequate maternal and early life nutrition. In fact, there are broader efforts already in place for accelerating knowledge of genome-to-phenome associations in livestock that are applying core "omics" technologies including RNA-seq.[1] These efforts are instrumental for the study of chromatin architecture, transcription

The authors have nothing to disclose.
Department of Animal Sciences, Division of Nutritional Sciences, University of Illinois, 1207 West Gregory Drive, Urbana, IL 61801, USA
* Corresponding author.
E-mail address: jloor@illinois.edu

factor binding site identification, analysis of histone modification marks, methylation, and genome conformation in livestock. This article has been divided into sections concerned with (1) epigenetic mechanisms, (2) maternal epigenetics and cellular mechanisms, and (3) epigenetic mechanisms in the offspring. Emphasis is placed in not only describing general aspects, but also discussing available data in livestock species linking nutrition and epigenetics (**Table 1**).

EPIGENETICS MECHANISMS
Chromatin Architecture Remodeling (Euchromatin, Heterochromatin)

Normally, DNA is tightly coiled around histones, highly alkaline proteins found in eukaryotic cell nuclei that package and order the DNA into structural units (eg, nucleosomes). This forms the condensed heterochromatin rendering genes transcriptionally inactivated. DNA can then open to form euchromatin, a lightly packed form of chromatin, for gene expression to take place. This so-called chromatin remodeling can operate both at a local and at a global level: locally it can affect single gene expression, and globally it can change the accessibility of chromosome domains or even entire chromosomes.[2] In eukaryotes, the fundamental unit of chromosome folding is the nucleosome; it is formed by a segment of DNA about 146 bp long wrapped around 8 histone proteins.[3] The transcriptional machinery cannot access the DNA fragment of the nucleosome when they are tightly packed in heterochromatin form. Chromatin remodeling is orchestrated by multiple epigenetic processes: some directly modify the DNA molecule itself (eg, DNA methylation), whereas others relate to modifications of chromatin-associated proteins (eg, posttranslational histone modification).

DNA Methylation

DNA methylation is one of the best-characterized and major epigenetic modifications found in most eukaryotes. It is essential for normal development and it is involved in various biological processes, such as gene expression regulation, genomic imprinting, X chromosome inactivation, the suppression of repetitive elements, and carcinogenesis.[4]

Molecular and genetic studies in mammals have revealed that the DNA of vertebrate animals can be covalently modified by methylation of the cytosine base in the dinucleotide sequence 5′CpG3′, a cytosine and guanine separated by a phosphate that links the 2 nucleotides together in DNA.[5] In mammals, DNA methylation patterns are established during embryonic development by de novo methylating enzymes called Dnmt3a and Dnmt3b, and they are maintained by a Dnmt1-mediated copying mechanism when cells divide.[6] The heritability of DNA methylation patterns provides an epigenetic marking of the genome that is stable through multiple cell divisions and, thus, constitutes a form of cellular memory. For this reason, historically, DNA methylation has represented the archetypal mechanism of epigenetic inheritance. The methyl moiety of methyl cytosine resides in the major groove of the DNA helix where many DNA-binding proteins make contact with DNA. Thus, methylation likely exerts its effect by attracting or repelling various DNA-binding proteins. A family of proteins known as methyl-CpG binding domain proteins are attracted to and bind DNA-containing methylated CpG dinucleotides[7] before recruiting repressor complexes to methylated promoter regions, thereby contributing to transcriptional silencing. Conversely, regions of CpG methylation are known to prevent the protein binding of certain transcription factors, thereby preventing transcription.[7]

Profiling DNA methylation maps across the genome is important for understanding DNA methylation changes that occur during development and in disease phenotypes.

Table 1
Alterations in epigenetic marks in response to nutrition in livestock species

Treatment	Study Type	Experimental Design	Supplementation Period	Organ	Epigenetic Effect	Model and Reference
Epigenetic mark: methylation						
High-concentrate diet	In vivo	High-concentrate diet (60% concentrate + 40% forage) vs low-concentrate diet (40% concentrate + 60% forage)	Daily during mid-lactation (106–232 d in milk)	Liver	↑ Methylation of *SCD* ↓ Methylation of immune-related genes (*TLR4, LBP, HP, SAA3P, CSN1S1*)	Dairy cows[45,46]
Energy restriction	In vivo	Maternal dietary energy level: 85% (low) vs 140% (high) of metabolizable energy requirements	Daily supply during mid-to-late pregnancy (147–247 d of pregnancy) in beef cows	Fetal skeletal muscle	↑ Methylation of *IGF2*	Beef fetus[43]
Methionine	In vivo	Rumen-protected methionine (0.09% of the diet dry matter)	Daily supply during the peripartal period (−21 to +30 d in milk)	Liver	↑ Methylation of *PPARA* ↓ Global DNA methylation	Peripartal dairy cows[47]
Methionine or choline supply	In vivo	Rumen-protected methionine (0.08% of the diet dry matter) or rumen-protected choline (60 g/d)	Daily supply during the peripartal period (−21 to +30 d in milk)	Embryonic cells	↓ Global DNA methylation in response to maternal methionine supply ↔ Global DNA methylation in response to maternal choline supply	Dairy cow embryos at 6.5 d of pregnancy[48]
Nutrient restriction	In vivo	Maternal 50% nutrient-restricted diet vs 100% diet	10 mo	Offspring liver	↓ Global DNA Methylation	Male sheep offspring[44]

(continued on next page)

Table 1
(continued)

Energy source	In vitro	Corn diet vs hay diet while maintaining equivalent metabolizable energy	Daily supply during mid-pregnancy (67–132 d of pregnancy)	Skeletal muscle	↑ Methylation of lincRNA in response to corn ↓ Methylation of genes play a role in lipid metabolism, muscle growth, and insulin signaling: *LPAR3, PLIN4, PLIN5, NBEA,* and *SREBF1* in response to corn	Sheep fetus[42]
Vitamin B$_{12}$	In vitro	Oocytes were matured in vitro in medium supplemented with 200 pmol/L vitamin B$_{12}$	24-h incubation	Embryonic cells	↑ Global DNA methylation	Sheep embryo[49]
Feed restriction	In vivo	Maternal feed restriction during the periconceptional period; 2.1 kg diet/gilt vs 3 kg diet/gilt	Daily supply from the onset of estrus and throughout natural mating until 9 d of pregnancy	Endometrium and entire embryos at 16 d of gestation	In endometrium: ↑ Methylation of *ACP5, RGS12* and *TLR3* ↓ Methylation of *EDNRB* In embryos: ↑ Methylation of *ADIPOR2* and *DNMT1*	Porcine endometrium and embryos[50]
Vitamin C	In vitro	250 µmol/L L-ascorbic acid	Incubation for 44 h	Oocytes at the final stage of maturation	↑ Methylation of *TET2* ↓ Methylation of *DNMT3A*	Porcine oocytes[51]

Methyl donors	In vivo	Maternal supply with betaine (3 g/kg diet) + choline (400 mg/kg diet) + folic acid (15 mg/kg diet) + vitamin B$_{12}$ (150 μg/kg diet)	Daily supply from mating until delivery	Offspring liver	↑ Methylation of IGF1	Offspring pigs at 110 kg body weight[52]
Methyl donors	In vivo	Maternal supply with betaine (3 g/kg diet) + choline (400 mg/kg diet) + folic acid (15 mg/kg diet) + vitamin B$_{12}$ (150 μg/kg diet)	Daily supply throughout gestation	Offspring small intestine	↑ Methylation of SLC15A1	Offspring pigs at birth[53]
Methionine	In vivo	30% methionine > basal diet methionine content	Daily supply for 160 d	Skeletal muscle	↑ Methylation of MSTN	Piglets at weaning, 21 d of age[54]
Betaine	In vivo	Maternal supply with betaine (3 g/kg diet)	Daily supply throughout gestation	Offspring liver	↑ Methylation of GALK1	Male piglets at birth[55]
Manganese	In vivo	100, 50, and 10 mg manganese/kg diet from 2 sources: manganese oxide (MnO) and manganese nanoparticles (NP-Mn$_2$O$_3$)	Daily supply for 98 d	Blood	↔ Global DNA methylation in response to NP-Mn$_2$O$_3$ compared with MnO; ↓ Global DNA methylation in response to 50 and 100 mg/kg compared with 10 mg manganese/kg	Turkey hens[56]

(continued on next page)

Table 1
(continued)

Methionine or betaine	In vivo	1.2 g methionine/kg diet or 0.6 g betaine/kg diet	Daily supply for 50 d	Liver	↓ Methylation of LOC106032502, a key gene in amino acid transport and metabolism	Male geese at 21 d of age[57]
Methionine	In vivo	L-Methionine, DL-methionine, and methionine analogue, DL-2-hydroxy-4-(methylthio) butanoic acid to provide 0.22% methionine equivalent	Daily supply for 32 d	Liver	↔ Global DNA methylation	Male Cobb-500 broilers at 3 d of age[58]
Zinc	In ovo	2 Zinc (Zn) source (inorganic Zn sulfate and organic Zn-lysine) × 2 Zn level (50 and 100 µg Zn/egg)	One-time injection at early stage of incubation (on E9–10)	Liver	↔ Global DNA methylation	Broiler breeder eggs[59]
Polysaccharides	In vivo	Parental 10 g Astragalus Polysaccharides/kg diet	Daily to Avein breeder cocks from 0 to 40 weeks of age	Offspring spleen	↔ Methylation of MyD88 and TICAM1	Offspring broilers at 14 d of age[60]
Betaine	In vivo	Maternal 0.5% betaine-supplemented diet	Daily to hens for 30 d	Offspring hypothalamus	↓ Methylation of SREBF1, SREBP-2 and APOA1	Offspring broilers at 56 d of age[61]
Betaine	In vivo	Maternal 0.5% betaine-supplemented diet	Daily to hens for 28 d	Offspring liver	↑ Methylation of DIO1	Offspring broilers at 56 d of age[62]

Betaine	In ovo	One-time injection	2.5 mg betaine/egg	Hypothalamus	↓ Methylation of HMGCR, ABCA1 and ACAT1 ↑ Methylation of LDLR	Male offspring broilers at 64 d of age[63]
Betaine	In ovo	One-time injection	2.5 mg betaine/egg	Liver	↑ Methylation of NR1H3 and CYP27A1	Male offspring broilers at 56 d of age[64]

Epigenetic mark: acetylation

High-concentrate diet	In vivo	Daily supply for 6 wk	(1) high-concentrate corn straw (HCS) diet (65% concentrate + 35% corn straw); (2) low-concentrate corn straw (LCS) diet (46% concentrate + 54% corn straw); (3) low-concentrate mixed forage (LMF) diet (46% concentrate + 54% mixed forage)	Mammary gland	↓ Acetylation in HCS cows	Midlactation dairy cows[65]
Zinc	In ovo	One-time injection at early stage of incubation (on E9–10)	Two Zinc (Zn) sources (inorganic Zn sulfate and organic Zn-lysine) × 2 Zn levels (50 and 100 μg Zn/egg)	Liver	↔ Acetylation of MT4 in response to Zn injection ↑ Acetylation of EHMT2 in response to organic Zn compared with inorganic Zn	Broiler breeder eggs[59]

Abbreviations: ABCA1, ATP binding cassette subfamily A member 1; *ACAT1*, acetyl-CoA acetyltransferase 1; *ACP5*, acid phosphatase 5, tartrate resistant; *ADIPOR2*, adiponectin receptor 2; *APOA1*, apolipoprotein A1; *CSN1S1*, casein alpha S1; *CYP27A1*, cytochrome P450 family 27 subfamily A member 1; *DIO1*, iodothyronine deiodinase 1; *DNMT1*, DNA methyltransferase 1; *DNMT3A*, DNA methyltransferase 3 alpha; *EDNRB*, endothelin receptor type B; *EHMT2*, euchromatic histone lysine methyltransferase 2; *GALK1*, galactokinase 1; *HMGCR*, 3-hydroxy-3-methylglutaryl-CoA reductase; *HP*, haptoglobin; *IGF1*, insulin-like growth factor 1; *IGF2*, insulin-like growth factor 2; *LBP*, lipopolysaccharide binding protein; *LDLR*, low-density lipoprotein receptor; *MSTN*, myostatin; *MT4*, metallothionein 4; *MYD88*, myeloid differentiation primary response 88; *NR1H3*, nuclear receptor subfamily 1 group H member 3; *PPARA*, peroxisome proliferator activated receptor alpha; *RGS12*, regulator of G protein signaling 12; *RPS6KB1*, ribosomal protein S6 kinase B1; *SAA3P*, serum amyloid A3, pseudogene; *SCD*, stearoyl-CoA desaturase; *SLC15A1*, solute carrier family 15 member 1; *SREBF1*, sterol regulatory element binding transcription factor 1; *TET2*, tet methylcytosine dioxygenase 2; *TICAM1*, toll-like receptor adaptor molecule 1; *TLR3*, toll like receptor 3; *TLR4*, toll-like receptor 4.

Genome-wide DNA methylation maps of many organisms including human, chicken, rat, Arabidopsis, rice, and silkworm have been published.[8] The methylation pattern of cattle has also been recently reported in placenta,[8] blastocysts,[9] and sperm.[10]

Although DNA methylation patterns can be transmitted from cell to cell, they are not permanent. In fact, changes in DNA methylation patterns can occur throughout the life of an individual. Some changes can be a physiologic response to environmental changes, whereas others might be associated with a pathologic process such as oncogenic transformation or cellular aging. DNA methylation marks can be removed by either an active demethylation mechanism involving a family of DNA hydroxylases called Tet proteins or a passive demethylation process by inhibition of the maintenance methyltransferase, Dnmt1, during cell divisions.[4]

Posttranscriptional Histone Modifications

Histones are proteins that package and order eukaryotic genomes into chromatin, which play an important role in epigenetic regulation with varying covalent modifications. Histones mainly contain 5 families: H1, H2A, H2B, H3, H4, and H5.[11] All histones are subject to a variety of posttranscriptional modifications, of which the most studied are acetylation and methylation.

Histone acetylation usually takes place on multiple lysine residues located within their N-terminal termini, primarily of histone 3 and 4.[12] Histone acetylation and deacetylation is mediated by opposing practices of histone acetyl transferases and histone deacetylases (HDACs), respectively.[13] The histone acetyl transferases are believed to relax the chromatin structure and allow access for transcription factors, thereby promoting gene expression.[14] Conversely, HDAC promote tighter DNA–histone interaction and repress transcriptional activity.[14] Histone methylation is generally involved in monomethylation, dimethylation, or trimethylation of lysine residues of histone 3, or arginine residues of histone 2A, 3, and 4.[12] The consequences of histone methylation for gene expression are complex, because methylation may have opposite consequences depending on localization and number of methyl groups.

Other histone modifications have also been observed. Histone phosphorylation, ubiquitination, and ADP-ribosylation complete the spectrum of the 5 known posttranscriptional histone modification, together with the aforementioned acetylation and methylation.[15] Respectively, they alter histone proteins and their functions by linking a phosphate group, 1 or more ubiquitin molecules, and target the histone for degradation, or by adding 1 or more ADP-ribose moieties. Histone phosphorylation predominantly takes place during cellular response to DNA damage, when phosphorylated histone 2A demarcates large chromatin domains around the site of DNA breakage.[16] However, multiple studies have also shown that histone phosphorylation plays crucial roles in chromatin remodeling linked to other nuclear processes.[16] Histone 2A was the first protein identified to be modified by ubiquitin in cells, and we currently know that histones 2A and 2B are 2 of the most abundant ubiquitinated proteins in the nucleus.[17] Their ubiquitination plays critical roles in many processes in the nucleus, including transcription, maintenance of chromatin structure, and DNA repair.[17] Similarly to phosphorylation and ubiquitination, histone ADP-ribosylation is involved in DNA repair, replication, and transcription.[18]

MATERNAL EPIGENETICS AND CELLULAR MECHANISMS
Preimplantation Embryo

The initial period of preimplantation development depends mainly on maternal proteins and messenger RNA (mRNA) stored in the oocyte cytoplasm.[19] The transition from maternal to embryonic control of development includes the degradation of maternal products and zygotic genome activation (ZGA)[20] characterized by massive transcription of the embryonic genome that is important for further embryonic development.[21] To ensure a proper ZGA, a complete epigenetic remodeling is required during early development.[22] The paternal genome undergoes a remarkable transformation in the egg cytoplasm, where remodeling of sperm chromatin through removal of protamines and replacement by histones is closely followed by genome-wide demethylation, which is complete before DNA replication commences.[22]

Few histone methyltransferases control the correct maintenance of the epigenome during epigenetic remodeling of embryos,[21] these include euchromatic histone lysine methyltransferase 1 (EHMT1/2), histone-lysine N-methyltransferase 1 (SUV39H1/H2/SETDB1), and isocitrate dehydrogenase (NADP(+))2 (EDH2), which regulate the methylation of histone H3K9 dimethylation (H3K9me2), histone H3 lysine 9 trimethylation (H3K9me3), and histone H3 lysine 9 or 27 trimethylation (H3K927me3), respectively.[21] From the transcription level, lysine demethylases (KDM), enzymes responsible for removal of the methylation marks from H3K4, H3K9, and H3K27, are likely involved in the regulation of the ZGA transition.[23] During subsequent phases of development, despite the presence of DNMT1 and DNMT3A, the abundance of DNMT3B plays a major role in regulating methylation levels.[24,25] The role of these genes/proteins is underscored by the fact that DNMT3A, DNMT3B, and DNMT3L are required for increasing differentially methylated regions of bovine imprinted genes during oocyte growth.[26]

Placenta

In rodents and humans, maternal nutrition and environmental stressors such as smoking and alcohol consumption during pregnancy affect offspring growth and development through epigenetic effects.[27] Whereas the embryonic parental epigenome, acquired from both parental gametes during fertilization, undergoes major reprogramming during early development, in utero maternal epigenetic effects take place in the periimplantation period. Subsequently, the placenta acquires an important role after implantation. From its earliest stages until the end of pregnancy, the placenta is of paramount importance for the intrauterine development and growth of the fetus. It is responsible for the establishment of a tight contact between mother and conceptus, enabling the exchange of gas, nutrients, and waste products, with roles in immune response and hormone secretion among other important physiologic functions.[28] Disruption of placentation has negative effects on both mother and fetus.[29] Furthermore, a significant factor in placental development and function is epigenetic regulation, with DNA methylation, histone modifications, noncoding RNA, and genomic imprinting having important roles.[30]

Maternal health status, plane of nutrition, or exposure to exogenous contaminants typically found in foods can elicit epigenetic effects in placenta. For instance, different methylation profiles were detected in placenta from women afflicted by gestational diabetes.[31] Maternal glycemia at the second and third trimesters of pregnancy also is related to variations in placental DNA methylation levels at the PR domain containing 16 (PRDM16), bone morphogenetic protein 7 (BMP7), and peroxisome proliferator-activated receptor gamma coactivator 1-alpha (PPARGC1A).[32] Work with rodents also has underscored a link between maternal obesity and histone modifications in placental labyrinth.[33] Compared with normal mice, tissue from obese animals had greater mRNA abundance of the lysine acetyltransferases Kat1, Kat3, and Kat13b, whereas expression of lysine methyltransferase (Ehmt1) and HDACs (Hdac3 and Hdac10).[33] These data underscore the potential for nutritional management of livestock to control the expression of genes related to energy metabolism, glucose homeostasis, and insulin signaling via changes in DNA methylation.

Imprinted genes, which are epigenetically regulated, are highly expressed in placenta and usually are lacking in nonplacental organisms.[22] Mutant *Dnmt1* resulted in the biallelic expression of certain genes in the regulating domains of insulin-like growth factor 2 (*Igf2*), small nuclear ribonucleoprotein polypeptide N (*Snrpn*), and paternally expressed 3 (*Peg3*), whereas genes in the *Kcnq1* domain were less sensitive to absence of *Dnmt1* suggesting that DNA methylation plays a critical role in imprinting.[34] The relevance of these data to livestock is underscored by the fact that an abundance of imprinted genes such as *IGF2R* and imprinted maternally expressed transcript (H19) along with *DNMT3a* and maternally expressed 8 (*MEG8*) in skeletal muscle of beef cattle offspring was altered by maternal plane of dietary energy during the last half of gestation.[35]

EPIGENETIC MECHANISMS IN THE OFFSPRING

In rodents and humans, DNA methylation and histone acetylation can be modified by dietary compounds.[36,37] In livestock, both in vivo and in vitro studies indicate that nutrition can induce epigenetic changes in different tissues such as liver, skeletal muscle, mammary gland, and ruminal epithelium (see **Table 1**). In the context of mechanisms, DNA methylation has been the most studied in livestock, with nutrients such as methionine, folate, betaine, and choline or the total supply of nutrients (ie, overfeeding or restricting) to the mother being the main factors of interest.[38]

One of the first studies with ruminants attempting to link maternal diet and mRNA profiles in the fetus was that of Peñagaricano and colleagues[39] in which the level of fiber (F), starch (S), or F plus protein plus fat (FPF) of the dam was changed to assess its effect on skeletal muscle and adipose mRNA profiles. Because all diets were isoenergetic, the investigators could assess the direct role of these macronutrients on the developing embryo. Both F and FPF compared with S induced transcriptome-wide changes in genes related to myogenesis and muscle differentiation. Likewise, feeding FPF relative to S caused marked alterations in the adipose tissue transcriptome associated with adipogenesis, chromatin biology, and metabolic processes among others.[39] Although this study did not assess epigenetic changes per se, another study using the same experimental design revealed greater methylation status of CpG islands of the imprinted genes *IGF2R* and *H19* in the longissimus muscle of fetuses from dams fed F and FPF compared with S.[40] It was proposed that a greater supply of amino acids (and methyl donors) in the F and FPF diets relative to S was partly responsible for the greater degree of methylation.

Because of their well-established role as methyl donors, there is ongoing interest on understanding whether the supply of dietary vitamin B_{12}, folate, methionine, betaine, or choline could impact epigenetic mechanisms in livestock. In one of the first studies of its kind, restricting the dietary supply of vitamin B_{12}, folate, and methionine within normal physiologic ranges during the periconceptional period in female sheep had no effect on birth weight, but induced greater body and fat mass deposition in the adult male offspring.[41] Such physiologic changes were associated with widespread alterations in DNA methylation of the fetal liver. A link between the supply of methionine, choline, and folate during mid-to-late pregnancy in sheep and fetal longissimus muscle DNA methylation and transcriptome profiles was recently confirmed.[42] That study revealed a number of distinct changes in the number of differentially methylated regions when dams were fed a greater level of methionine plus choline versus greater folate. The absence of phenotype data precluded a more thorough evaluation of the physiologic outcomes as a result of epigenetic changes.

Maternal feed restriction during pregnancy induces epigenetic changes in the fetus and offspring through the alteration of DNA methylation. In a recent study, Paradis and colleagues[43] showed that restricting total nutrient supply from mid to late pregnancy (feeding at 85% vs 140% of total metabolizable energy requirements) in beef cows induced hypermethylation of CpG in the differentially methylated region 2 of *IGF2* without altering the mRNA abundance of the gene in fetal skeletal muscle.[43] In another study, Chadio and colleagues[44] observed that maternal feed restriction in pregnant ewes (50% nutrient-restriction from days 0 to 30, or from days 31 to 100 of pregnancy) did not affect body weight of male offspring at birth or at 10 months of age, whereas feed restriction during pregnancy decreased liver weight and hepatic DNA methylation in the offspring.[44]

Work in swine has highlighted how brief periods of undernutrition during key stages of pregnancy can alter the epigenome of the offspring. An important biological step during early development is the epigenetic maternal imprinting after the embryo epigenome undergoes a major reset to allow for a proper ZGA. Between the blastocyst stage and implantation, the uterine endometrium can alter the embryo methylome. When gilts were underfed during the periconceptional period (from days 0 to 9 of pregnancy), methylation was responsible for changes in mRNA abundance in both the mother endometrium and the embryonic tissues.[49] The affected genes span functions associated with immune response, uterine–embryo iron transport, metabolic homeostasis, and methylation itself.

PERSPECTIVES

In the context of physiologic responses that determine the growth, development, and health status of livestock, the role of epigenetics and the underlying cellular mechanisms it affects remain to be fully elucidated. Although recent work with pigs, cattle, and small ruminants has provided evidence that maternal dietary energy level, carbohydrate type, or intestinal supply of methyl donors can elicit molecular changes in tissues of the embryo, fetus, or neonate, there are few data linking epigenetics with biochemical and physiologic outcomes. Therefore, future efforts linking the epigenome with physiologic and developmental outcomes offer exciting opportunities for in-depth discoveries that can impact efficiency of nutrient use and well-being of livestock.

ACKNOWLEDGMENTS

Ahmed Elolimy is a recipient of a PhD fellowship from the Higher Education Ministry of Egypt to perform his studies at the University of Illinois (Urbana). Yusheng Liang is a recipient of a PhD fellowship from the China Scholarship Council (Beijing) to perform his studies at the University of Illinois (Urbana).

REFERENCES

1. Loor JJ, Vailati-Riboni M, McCann JC, et al. Triennial lactation symposium: nutrigenomics in livestock: systems biology meets nutrition. J Anim Sci 2015;93(12): 5554–74.
2. De Majo F, Calore M. Chromatin remodelling and epigenetic state regulation by non-coding RNAs in the diseased heart. Noncoding RNA Res 2018;3(1):20–8.
3. Grewal SI, Moazed D. Heterochromatin and epigenetic control of gene expression. Science 2003;301(5634):798–802.
4. Li E, Zhang Y. DNA methylation in mammals. Cold Spring Harb Perspect Biol 2014;6(5):a019133.

5. Rothbart SB, Strahl BD. Interpreting the language of histone and DNA modifications. Biochim Biophys Acta 2014;1839(8):627–43.

6. Portela A, Esteller M. Epigenetic modifications and human disease. Nat Biotechnol 2010;28(10):1057–68.

7. Du Q, Luu PL, Stirzaker C, et al. Methyl-CpG-binding domain proteins: readers of the epigenome. Epigenomics 2015;7(6):1051–73.

8. Su J, Wang Y, Xing X, et al. Genome-wide analysis of DNA methylation in bovine placentas. BMC Genomics 2014;15:12.

9. Salilew-Wondim D, Fournier E, Hoelker M, et al. Genome-wide DNA methylation patterns of bovine blastocysts developed in vivo from embryos completed different stages of development in vitro. PLoS One 2015;10(11):e0140467.

10. Zhou Y, Connor EE, Bickhart DM, et al. Comparative whole genome DNA methylation profiling of cattle sperm and somatic tissues reveals striking hypomethylated patterns in sperm. Gigascience 2018;7(5):1–13.

11. Banks DD, Gloss LM. Equilibrium folding of the core histones: the H3-H4 tetramer is less stable than the H2A-H2B dimer. Biochemistry 2003;42(22):6827–39.

12. Ye J, Wu W, Li Y, et al. Influences of the gut microbiota on DNA methylation and histone modification. Dig Dis Sci 2017;62(5):1155–64.

13. Dose A, Liokatis S, Theillet FX, et al. NMR profiling of histone deacetylase and acetyl-transferase activities in real time. ACS Chem Biol 2011;6(5):419–24.

14. Mahgoub M, Monteggia LM. A role for histone deacetylases in the cellular and behavioral mechanisms underlying learning and memory. Learn Mem 2014; 21(10):564–8.

15. Strahl BD, Allis CD. The language of covalent histone modifications. Nature 2000; 403(6765):41–5.

16. Rossetto D, Avvakumov N, Cote J. Histone phosphorylation: a chromatin modification involved in diverse nuclear events. Epigenetics 2012;7(10):1098–108.

17. Cao J, Yan Q. Histone ubiquitination and deubiquitination in transcription, DNA damage response, and cancer. Front Oncol 2012;2:26.

18. Messner S, Hottiger MO. Histone ADP-ribosylation in DNA repair, replication and transcription. Trends Cell Biol 2011;21(9):534–42.

19. Tadros W, Lipshitz HD. The maternal-to-zygotic transition: a play in two acts. Development 2009;136(18):3033–42.

20. Hamatani T, Carter MG, Sharov AA, et al. Dynamics of global gene expression changes during mouse preimplantation development. Dev Cell 2004;6(1): 117–31.

21. Ross PJ, Sampaio RV. Epigenetic remodeling in preimplantation embryos: cows are not big mice. Anim Reprod 2018;15(3):204–14.

22. Reik W, Dean W, Walter J. Epigenetic reprogramming in mammalian development. Science 2001;293(5532):1089–93.

23. Glanzner WG, Rissi VB, de Macedo MP, et al. Histone 3 lysine 4, 9, and 27 demethylases expression profile in fertilized and cloned bovine and porcine embryos. Biol Reprod 2018;98(6):742–51.

24. Golding MC, Williamson GL, Stroud TK, et al. Examination of DNA methyltransferase expression in cloned embryos reveals an essential role for Dnmt1 in bovine development. Mol Reprod Dev 2011;78(5):306–17.

25. Dobbs KB, Rodriguez M, Sudano MJ, et al. Dynamics of DNA methylation during early development of the preimplantation bovine embryo. PLoS One 2013;8(6): e66230.

26. O'Doherty AM, O'Shea LC, Fair T. Bovine DNA methylation imprints are established in an oocyte size-specific manner, which are coordinated with the expression of the DNMT3 family proteins. Biol Reprod 2012;86(3):67, 61-10.
27. Kitsiou-Tzeli S, Tzetis M. Maternal epigenetics and fetal and neonatal growth. Curr Opin Endocrinol Diabetes Obes 2017;24(1):43–6.
28. Rossant J, Cross JC. Placental development: lessons from mouse mutants. Nat Rev Genet 2001;2(7):538.
29. Nelissen EC, van Montfoort AP, Dumoulin JC, et al. Epigenetics and the placenta. Hum Reprod Update 2010;17(3):397–417.
30. Maccani MA, Marsit CJ. Epigenetics in the placenta. Am J Reprod Immunol 2009; 62(2):78–89.
31. Finer S, Mathews C, Lowe R, et al. Maternal gestational diabetes is associated with genome-wide DNA methylation variation in placenta and cord blood of exposed offspring. Hum Mol Genet 2015;24(11):3021–9.
32. Côté S, Gagné-Ouellet V, Guay S-P, et al. PPARGC1α gene DNA methylation variations in human placenta mediate the link between maternal hyperglycemia and leptin levels in newborns. Clin Epigenetics 2016;8(1):72.
33. Panchenko PE, Voisin S, Jouin M, et al. Expression of epigenetic machinery genes is sensitive to maternal obesity and weight loss in relation to fetal growth in mice. Clin Epigenetics 2016;8(1):22.
34. Weaver JR, Sarkisian G, Krapp C, et al. Domain-specific response of imprinted genes to reduced DNMT1. Mol Cell Biol 2010;30(16):3916–28.
35. Wang X, Lan X, Radunz AE, et al. Maternal nutrition during pregnancy is associated with differential expression of imprinted genes and DNA methyltransferases in muscle of beef cattle offspring. J Anim Sci 2015;93(1):35–40.
36. Delage B, Dashwood RH. Dietary manipulation of histone structure and function. Annu Rev Nutr 2008;28:347–66.
37. Canani RB, Di Costanzo M, Leone L, et al. Epigenetic mechanisms elicited by nutrition in early life. Nutr Res Rev 2011;24(2):198–205.
38. Anderson OS, Sant KE, Dolinoy DC. Nutrition and epigenetics: an interplay of dietary methyl donors, one-carbon metabolism and DNA methylation. J Nutr Biochem 2012;23(8):853–9.
39. Penagaricano F, Wang X, Rosa GJ, et al. Maternal nutrition induces gene expression changes in fetal muscle and adipose tissues in sheep. BMC Genomics 2014; 15:1034.
40. Lan X, Cretney EC, Kropp J, et al. Maternal diet during pregnancy induces gene expression and DNA methylation changes in fetal tissues in sheep. Front Genet 2013;4:49.
41. Sinclair KD, Allegrucci C, Singh R, et al. DNA methylation, insulin resistance, and blood pressure in offspring determined by maternal periconceptional B vitamin and methionine status. Proc Natl Acad Sci U S A 2007;104(49):19351–6.
42. Namous H, Penagaricano F, Del Corvo M, et al. Integrative analysis of methylomic and transcriptomic data in fetal sheep muscle tissues in response to maternal diet during pregnancy. BMC Genomics 2018;19(1):123.
43. Paradis F, Wood KM, Swanson KC, et al. Maternal nutrient restriction in mid-to-late gestation influences fetal mRNA expression in muscle tissues in beef cattle. BMC Genomics 2017;18(1):632.
44. Chadio S, Kotsampasi B, Taka S, et al. Epigenetic changes of hepatic glucocorticoid receptor in sheep male offspring undernourished in utero. Reprod Fertil Dev 2017;29(10):1995–2004.

45. Xu TL, Seyfert HM, Shen XZ. Epigenetic mechanisms contribute to decrease stearoyl-CoA desaturase 1 expression in the liver of dairy cows after prolonged feeding of high-concentrate diet. J Dairy Sci 2018;101(3):2506–18.

46. Chang G, Zhang K, Xu T, et al. Epigenetic mechanisms contribute to the expression of immune related genes in the livers of dairy cows fed a high concentrate diet. PLoS One 2015;10(4):e0123942.

47. Osorio JS, Jacometo CB, Zhou Z, et al. Hepatic global DNA and peroxisome proliferator-activated receptor alpha promoter methylation are altered in peripartal dairy cows fed rumen-protected methionine. J Dairy Sci 2016;99(1):234–44.

48. Acosta DAV, Denicol AC, Tribulo P, et al. Effects of rumen-protected methionine and choline supplementation on the preimplantation embryo in Holstein cows. Theriogenology 2016;85(9):1669–79.

49. Zacchini F, Toschi P, Ptak GE. Cobalamin supplementation during in vitro maturation improves developmental competence of sheep oocytes. Theriogenology 2017;93:55–61.

50. Zglejc-Waszak K, Waszkiewicz EM, Franczak A. Periconceptional undernutrition affects the levels of DNA methylation in the peri-implantation pig endometrium and in embryos. Theriogenology 2019;123:185–93.

51. Yu XX, Liu YH, Liu XM, et al. Ascorbic acid induces global epigenetic reprogramming to promote meiotic maturation and developmental competence of porcine oocytes. Sci Rep 2018;8(1):6132.

52. Jin C, Zhuo Y, Wang J, et al. Methyl donors dietary supplementation to gestating sows diet improves the growth rate of offspring and is associating with changes in expression and DNA methylation of insulin-like growth factor-1 gene. J Anim Physiol Anim Nutr (Berl) 2018;102(5):1340–50.

53. Liu H, Wang J, Mou D, et al. Maternal methyl donor supplementation during gestation counteracts the bisphenol a-induced impairment of intestinal morphology, disaccharidase activity, and nutrient transporters gene expression in newborn and weaning pigs. Nutrients 2017;9(5) [pii:E423].

54. Li Y, Zhang H, Chen YP, et al. Effects of dietary l-methionine supplementation on the growth performance, carcass characteristics, meat quality, and muscular antioxidant capacity and myogenic gene expression in low birth weight pigs. J Anim Sci 2017;95(9):3972–83.

55. Cai D, Yuan M, Liu H, et al. Epigenetic and SP1-mediated regulation is involved in the repression of galactokinase 1 gene in the liver of neonatal piglets born to betaine-supplemented sows. Eur J Nutr 2017;56(5):1899–909.

56. Ognik K, Kozlowski K, Stepniowska A, et al. The effect of manganese nanoparticles on performance, redox reactions and epigenetic changes in turkey tissues. Animal 2018;1–8 [Epub ahead of print].

57. Yang Z, Yang HM, Gong DQ, et al. Transcriptome analysis of hepatic gene expression and DNA methylation in methionine- and betaine-supplemented geese (Anser cygnoides domesticus). Poult Sci 2018;97(10):3463–77.

58. Zhang S, Saremi B, Gilbert ER, et al. Physiological and biochemical aspects of methionine isomers and a methionine analogue in broilers. Poult Sci 2017;96(2):425–39.

59. Sun X, Lu L, Liao X, et al. Effect of in ovo zinc injection on the embryonic development and epigenetics-related indices of zinc-deprived broiler breeder eggs. Biol Trace Elem Res 2018;185(2):456–64.

60. Li Y, Lei X, Yin Z, et al. Transgenerational effects of paternal dietary Astragalus polysaccharides on spleen immunity of broilers. Int J Biol Macromol 2018;115:90–7.

61. Idriss AA, Hu Y, Hou Z, et al. Dietary betaine supplementation in hens modulates hypothalamic expression of cholesterol metabolic genes in F1 cockerels through modification of DNA methylation. Comp Biochem Physiol B Biochem Mol Biol 2018;217:14–20.
62. Hou Z, Sun Q, Hu Y, et al. Maternal betaine administration modulates hepatic type 1 iodothyronine deiodinase (Dio1) expression in chicken offspring through epigenetic modifications. Comp Biochem Physiol B Biochem Mol Biol 2018;218:30–6.
63. Idriss AA, Hu Y, Sun Q, et al. Prenatal betaine exposure modulates hypothalamic expression of cholesterol metabolic genes in cockerels through modifications of DNA methylation. Poult Sci 2017;96(6):1715–24.
64. Hu Y, Sun Q, Zong Y, et al. Prenatal betaine exposure alleviates corticosterone-induced inhibition of CYP27A1 expression in the liver of juvenile chickens associated with its promoter DNA methylation. Gen Comp Endocrinol 2017;246: 241–8.
65. Dong G, Qiu M, Ao C, et al. Feeding a high-concentrate corn straw diet induced epigenetic alterations in the mammary tissue of dairy cows. PLoS One 2014;9(9): e107659.

Overgrowth Syndrome

Yahan Li, BS, MS[a], Callum G. Donnelly, BVSc (Hons 1), DACT[b],
Rocío Melissa Rivera, BS, MS, PhD[a],*

KEYWORDS

- Overgrowth • Large offspring syndrome • Abnormal offspring syndrome
- Assisted reproduction • Spontaneous LOS

KEY POINTS

- Overgrowth syndromes (OGSs) refer to a heterogeneous group of conditions found in many species and can be divided into 2 categories based on phenotypes, namely generalized OGSs and localized/partial OGSs.
- Large offspring syndrome (LOS), also known as abnormal offspring syndrome, is a generalized congenital OGS in bovine most often observed in offspring conceived with the use of assisted reproductive technologies.
- Features of LOS include overgrowth, enlarged tongues, umbilical hernias, muscle and skeleton malformation, abnormal organ growth, allantois development defects, abnormal placental vasculature, and increased embryo or fetus death rates.
- Beckwith-Wiedemann syndrome is a human congenital overgrowth condition that emulates LOS. Both conditions are the result of epigenetic errors and have been characterized as loss-of-imprinting conditions.
- Fetal giants have been rarely recognized in naturally conceived calves that are born at normal gestation lengths, with the predominant abnormality absolute oversize. The authors propose that these calves represent spontaneous large offspring syndrome (S-LOS).

INTRODUCTION

Overgrowth syndromes (OGSs) refer to a heterogeneous group of conditions found in many species,[1–3] which show a common feature of excessive growth. According to the definitions used in humans, OGSs can be divided into 2 categories based on phenotypes: generalized OGSs and localized/partial OGSs.[1] Generalized OGSs often are characterized by a 2-3 standard deviations increase in overall growth parameters, including body weight, height, and head circumference.[4,5] On the other hand, localized/partial OGSs result in overgrowth in 1 or few organs or regions of the body.[6] OGS also can be characterized as congenital and/or postnatal according to the age

This work was supported by the Agriculture and Food Research Initiative Competitive Grant No. 2017-08953 from the USDA National Institute of Food and Agriculture.
[a] Division of Animal Sciences, University of Missouri, Columbia, MO 65211, USA; [b] Department of Medicine and Epidemiology, School of Veterinary Medicine, University of California, Davis, Davis, CA 95616, USA
* Corresponding author.
E-mail address: riverarm@missouri.edu

Vet Clin Food Anim 35 (2019) 265–276
https://doi.org/10.1016/j.cvfa.2019.02.007
0749-0720/19/© 2019 Elsevier Inc. All rights reserved.

when phenotypes present.[4,7–9] A greater risk of tumorigenesis is a shared feature of many OGSs found in humans.[1]

A generalized congenital OGS in bovine is known as LOS[2] (**Fig. 1**). LOS refers to a group of abnormal phenotypes occurring in bovine and ovine fetuses, placentas, and newborns produced by assisted reproductive technologies (ARTs). There are many ART-induced LOS calf reports from experimental studies.[10–14] Features of LOS include overgrowth, enlarged tongues, umbilical hernias, muscle and skeleton malformations, abnormal organ growth, allantois development defects, abnormal placental vasculature, and increased early embryo or fetus death rates.[15–18] LOS can affect the dam and cause death of the afflicted animal, bringing financial loss to producers. Although there is a lack of published reports providing the incidence of LOS in ART-produced offspring, this incidence has been reported as high as 10% (Rocio M. Rivera, personal communications, 2017).

CLINICAL FEATURES OF LARGE OFFSPRING SYNDROME

Macrosomia refers to increased body and limb size, the most commonly identified feature of LOS.[2,17,18] This increased size of body and limbs can be 2 times and 5 times greater than the average size at birth, respectively,[17] and the increased body size can be detected as early as the fifth week of gestation in cattle.[19] Increased skeletal lengths have been reported to be coupled with macrosomia.[14] Calves with macrosomia at birth, however, reach similar mature body weight as control animals.[20] Using the criteria for humans, birthweight greater than 2 times SD above the mean is defined as macrosomia.[21] Because LOS indicates overgrowth, it is easily taken for granted that macrosomia is a necessary feature. LOS, however, is not always characterized by overgrowth and thus sometimes referred to as abnormal offspring syndrome.[16]

Macroglossia (enlarged tongue) is a feature of LOS.[22] Severe macroglossia causes feeding and breathing difficulties. Abdominal wall defects, including omphalocele and umbilical hernia, also have been observed in LOS fetuses.[22] An omphalocele is the outward protrusion of abdominal organs through the umbilical cord, with the organs not being covered by skin but by membranes (ie, amnion, peritoneum, and Wharton jelly[23]). Omphalocele is a severe defect present at birth and requires immediate

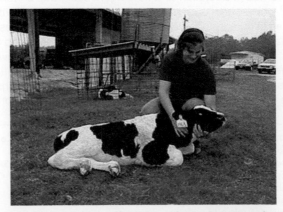

Fig. 1. ART-produced LOS. Large bull calf produced by in vitro procedures by Rocio Melissa Rivera while at the University of Florida. The picture was taken when the calf was 2 days of age. The calf weighed 98 kg at birth and died at 1 week of age as a result of complications relating to overgrowth, which included inability to stand up to suckle.

corrective surgeries. An umbilical hernia is a bulge of abdominal organs at the umbilicus, which is caused by incomplete closure of umbilical ring and is covered by skin.[24]

Organomegaly, the abnormal enlargement of organs, has been observed in heart, liver, and kidney of LOS calves.[14,25] In addition, placentomegaly, an abnormally enlarged placenta, has been found in cows carrying in vitro fertilization (IVF)–conceived fetuses.[18]

Other features, including increased incidence of hydrallantois,[12,15] increased gestation length,[26] increased dystocia rate,[27] ataxia/paresis,[28,29] and abnormal limbs combined with abnormal spine,[15] also have been observed in LOS calves.

ASSISTED REPRODUCTIVE TECHNOLOGIES AND LARGE OFFSPRING SYNDROME

In the late 1980s and 1990s, clinical epidemiologist Barker[30] suggested that the gestating maternal environment could have adverse consequences to the well-being of the offspring after birth. The phenomenon, which explains this permanent programming of the fetus, was named *fetal origins of adult disease* or the *Barker hypothesis*. The *developmental origins of health and disease hypothesis*, as the phenomenon is now known, propositions that the inherent developmental (genetic) program of an individual can be influenced by its environment, especially during critical periods of development, which can have significant long-term consequences for the well-being of the offspring during life. One artificial environment that has received much scientific attention for its potential to cause incorrect developmental programming to the resulting offspring in humans and livestock animals is ARTs.

ARTs refer to a series of laboratory techniques and procedures used to conceive offspring. ART procedures include oocyte retrieval from ovaries, in vitro oocyte maturation, IVF, embryo culture, and embryo transfer (ET). ARTs are used in cattle to improve genetic merit of the offspring in a shorted length of time compared with natural reproduction. Genetic merit is defined as the rank of an animal for its ability to produce superior offspring relative to other selection candidates (Purdue Extension—https://www.extension.purdue.edu/extmedia/nsif/nsif-8.pdf). In addition, ART can be used to produce genetically manipulated animals with improved production traits.[31]

Supplement of serum during in vitro embryo culture has been historically used to stimulate blastocyst formation.[32] Two experimental accounts suggest that serum can induce LOS in approximately 25% of ovine and bovine fetuses.[33,34] Adding fetal calf serum and bovine serum albumin during bovine embryo culture accelerates embryo development and improves blastocyst yield by day 6 but decreases embryo survival rate.[35,36] When comparing ovine embryos cultured with or without human serum supplements, bovine serum albumin, and amino acid supplements, increased body weight and gestation length in the human serum group were observed.[37] Coculture of embryos with various types of cells also has been used to increase blastocyst yield.[38] Similar to what has been found with serum supplementation in sheep, overgrowth[39,40] and increased gestation length[39] have been reported for ovine embryos that were cocultured with granulosa or oviduct epithelial cells. In addition, the size of the primary muscle fibers (which form during the first wave of myogenesis) and the ratio of secondary to primary fibers of the cocultured fetuses also were greater than in the controls, which indicate that hypertrophy of the primary fibers and hyperplasia of the secondary fibers are associated with the increased body weight observed in these fetuses.[40]

A SIMILAR OVERGROWTH SYNDROME OCCURS IN HUMANS

In humans, Beckwith-Wiedemann syndrome (BWS) (OMIM #130650), a human OGS, has phenotypical and molecular similarities to LOS. The most current report indicates an incidence of BWS in approximately 1/11,000 natural births.[41] BWS is a heterogeneous condition for which various phenotypic and (epi)genetic defects have been reported. Clinical features of BWS include macroglossia, abdominal wall defects (omphalocele/hernia/diastasis recti), lateralized overgrowth, childhood tumors (Wilms tumor and hepatoblastoma), neonatal hypoglycemia, macrosomia (large body size), ear malformations (creases/pits), facial nevus simplex (nevus flammeus or port-wine stain), and organomegaly.[21] The use of ARTs has been reported to increase the incidence of BWS by up to 10.7 times.[42,43]

MOLECULAR FINDINGS OF LARGE OFFSPRING SYNDROME AND BECKWITH-WIEDEMANN SYNDROME

The main molecular defects of BWS occur on human chromosome 11p15 (bovine = chromosome 29) and include defects in DNA methylation, incorrect expression of imprinted genes, changes of chromosomal contents, and gene mutations.[8,44–52] Among them, loss of imprinting caused by DNA methylation defects is the most frequently observed. DNA methylation (the addition of a methyl group [CH_3] to DNA) is an epigenetic mark involved in the control of gene expression. Genomic imprinting is an epigenetic phenomenon, which regulates parent-specific (ie, chromosome specific) gene expression of approximately 150 genes (ie, imprinted genes) in mammals.[53–56] These genes control growth and development of the fetus and the placenta and their expression is tightly regulated by a discrete region of differential DNA methylation known as the imprinting center (IC).[57] One of these ICs, namely, IC2 (also known as KvDMR1) is the most common genomic region affected by DNA methylation defects in BWS and LOS.[34] In a normal situation, the IC2 is methylated maternally inherited chromosome. This methylation state allows for the expression of the gene *KCNQ1OT1* from the paternal allele, which by attracting epigenetic modifiers, silences various flanking imprinted genes, including the cell cycle regulator *CDKN1C*.[58–60] The methylated state of the maternal chromosome orchestrates the expression of several genes involved in fetal and placental growth.[58–60] In LOS and BWS, imprinted gene expression regulated by the IC2 is lost as a result of loss of methylation of the maternal KvDMR1.[34,61–63]

ALTERATIONS IN GENE EXPRESSION

Alterations in imprinted and nonimprinted gene expression as a result of in vitro embryo production have been reported in numerous studies in bovine.[54,64–73] Different culture media and supplementation with serum cause transcript abundance changes of several developmentally important genes involved in cell-cell junctions, transport, RNA processing, and stress in bovine embryos.[64,65] The up-regulation of several developmentally important genes, including the imprinted gene *IGF1R*, have been suggested as early markers of LOS for bovine.[10] A 2-fold increase in expression of the imprinted fetal growth factor *IGF2* transcript can be detected in liver of day 70 bovine fetuses cultured in medium containing estrus cow serum when compared with the serum-restricted group.[74]

SPONTANEOUS LARGE OFFSPRING SYNDROME

Although LOS cases in bovine have only been reported associated with ARTs, LOS can occur spontaneously. Spontaneous maternal-fetal disproportion is the predominant cause of dystocia in beef cattle.[75] Several environmental and genetic factors cause this disparity and it is associated most commonly with first-calf heifers.[75,76]

Although calves in this scenario may be relatively large to the dam, they may not be oversized in absolute terms of population normals. In the human literature, neonates that are large for gestational age typically are above the 97th percentile for birthweight at delivery, although the definition varies slightly by condition.[77] Mechanistically, syndromes of overgrowth may be due to increased numbers of cells, hypertrophy, increases in the interstitium (such as fluid accumulation) or a combination of these conditions.[77] In humans, there are 2 broad categories of fetal OGSs. The first is those that are driven by the maternal environment, such as gestational diabetes, occurring in approximately 5% of all pregnancies.[78] Conditions, such as these, predominantly result in symmetric hypertrophy of fetal tissue, particularly adipose tissue. The second category is neonates that are affected by either spontaneous or inherited genetic mutations, such as BWS, Sotos syndrome, and Proteus syndrome, to name a few. Although these conditions are rare, they are becoming increasingly recognized, due to increased utilization of IVF techniques.[79] Spontaneous fetal oversize syndromes have not been well recognized in food animal species outside of neonates generated by ART.[2] For the purposes of this review, LOS can be categorized by conditions associated with prolonged gestation or those of normal gestational length.

Gestational length is relatively constant in cattle within breeds and environmental conditions, ranging from 280 days to 290 days.[80] Increasing gestational length within the normal range has been associated with larger birthweight.[76] Gestational length is moderately heritable and displays a gender bias, with male calves generally having longer gestational lengths than female calves.[76] A definition for post-term for cattle has not been established but is generally in excess of 300 days. Prolonged gestation has long been associated with a poor outcome for the resultant neonate.[81] Several breeds, including Ayrshire, Holstein Friesian, Guernsey, Jersey, Swedish Red and White, and Belgian Blue cattle, have been documented with pathologically prolonged gestation.[82–84] Prolonged gestation in these cases largely is secondary a to a dysfunctional hypothalamic-pituitary-adrenal axis, with the calf failing to initiate parturition. These conditions have included adenohypophyseal hypoplasia/aplasia, cerebellar hypoplasia, and adrenal hypoplasia. A genetic mutation has been suspected in many of these cases, with the mode of inheritance established but putative genetic mutations not. Infectious causes, such as Akabane virus, bluetongue virus, and bovine viral diarrhea virus, and toxic causes, such as ingestion of *Veratrum californicum*, also may result in prolonged gestation due to dysfunction of the hypothalamic-pituitary axis.[85] Prolonged gestation alone, however, does not always result in fetal oversize, with this syndrome only identified in Holstein Friesian, Swedish Red and White, and Ayrshire cattle.[2,76] Calves affected by overgrowth, commonly referred to as fetal giants, characteristically have long teeth, hair coats, and toes and otherwise appear normal. These calves have been reported to weigh between 59 kg and 98 kg. Typically, these calves are delivered after induction of parturition and almost invariably necessitate caesarean section. The traits that produce prolonged gestation and fetal oversize largely are incompatible with postnatal life and these calves rarely survive for more than 24 hours.

Although rare, fetal giants also have been recognized in calves that are born at normal gestation lengths, with the predominant abnormality absolute oversize. No specific descriptions of these calves have been made, other than Roberts[86] regarding any calf over 59 kg at birth to be a fetal giant. Despite reported by clinicians and producers, there are, to the authors' knowledge, no published descriptions of fetal giant LOS outside that of calves produced by IVF.

SPONTANEOUS LARGE OFFSPRING SYNDROME: CASE STUDIES

Three cases of S-LOS are illustrated in **Fig. 2**. The first calf was a purebred male Holstein Friesian calf that was delivered via caesarean section at 293 days of gestation. The calf weighed 83 kg at birth with the combined weight of the fetal membranes 12.7 kg. The calf had an appropriate hair coat, erupted teeth, and normal eponychium. The calf was proportionate with no obvious musculoskeletal defects. The calf did have an enlarged tongue (macroglossia) and large umbilical hernia

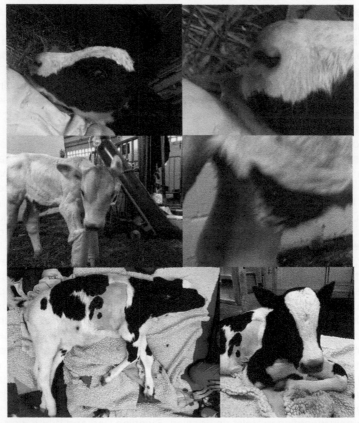

Fig. 2. Spontaneous LOS. Case 1 (*top left and right*)—a post-term 86-kg (normal birth at birth = 40–50 kg) Holstein bull calf was delivered by emergency cesarean section due to dystocia. The calf was macrosomic and had a marked omphalocele and macroglossia (*top right*). The calf was mentally inappropriate and was euthanized at 1 day of age. Immunohistochemistry of the anterior pituitary and hypothalamus could not demonstrate an aberration that could explain the macrosomia. Case 2 (*middle left and right*)—a preterm 63-kg Brown Swiss heifer (normal weight at birth approximately 45 kg) calf was delivered by planned cesarean section. The cow was referred for her large size approximately 2 weeks prior to being term. The calf was mentally appropriate at delivery and had an omphalocele and bilateral flexural deformities of the front metacarpophalangeal joint. The omphalocele was corrected surgically (*middle right*) and the flexural deformities by splints and physical therapy. The calf was discharged in good health and apparently is still performing well. Case 3 (*bottom left and right*)—1-day-old Holstein Friesian calf showing typical signs associated with LOS, including absolute macrosomia, omphalocele, and asymmetry of the pinna. The calf presented in respiratory distress and was later euthanized.

(omphalocele). The calf was unable to nurse due to the enlarged tongue and was humanely euthanized. Imaging of the brain by MRI and detailed necropsy definitively ruled out a structural alteration of the hypothalamus or pituitary or adrenal glands. The second calf was a female purebred Brown Swiss calf that was delivered at 283 days of gestation. The dam was initially presented due to concern for a hydrops condition with perceived overdistension of the abdomen at approximately 278 days of gestation. Based on palpation and transabdominal ultrasound, a hydrops condition was considered unlikely; however, the calf appeared very large. The calf was delivered by elective caesarean section after induction of parturition with cloprostenol and dexamethasone 40 hours prior to surgery. The viable calf weighed 63 kg at birth, with the fetal membranes unable to be weighed due to retention. The calf had small umbilical hernia and marked carpal contracture but was otherwise vigorous and healthy. The calf's legs were treated with splints and it was discharged at 10 days of age.

Although the definitive reason for fetal oversize has yet to be identified in these calves, it is strongly suspected that these calves represent S-LOS. After the identification of these 2 calves, other large-for-gestational-age calves not generated by IVF have been investigated and have been shown to possess the same epimutation as IVF-generated large offspring calves. This strongly emulates the analogous human condition BWS.[79]

Epigenetic conditions should be considered in cases of fetal gigantism where aberrations of gestational length have been excluded. At this time, risk factors have not been established and the occurrence of such calves is sporadic.

CONCLUDING REMARKS

The first ART calf was reported by Brackett and colleagues in 1982,[87] whereas the fact that ARTs can induce the birth of abnormally large calves was first documented in the 1990s.[11] Even though many reports have been published and almost 30 years have passed since the first LOS report, it is not yet possible to predict which embryos are molecularly programmed to suffer LOS, because the etiology of the syndrome is not known. Further, as Dr John F. Hasler states in a recent review of the ET industry, "there is a lack of peer-reviewed published data describing the current status of LOS problems in the commercial ET-IVP [embryo transfer - in vitro production] industry."[88] Therefore, it is difficult to calculate what the current incidence of LOS is and how much producers are affected. As discussed previously, off-the-record conversations have stated that 10% LOS in some practices is not unusual. For obvious reasons, the authors do not believe that such numbers will ever be published but hope to be able to provide information that may be used by ET companies and others using ART embryos in their practices to identify embryos molecularly programmed to suffer LOS prior to transfer.

Perinatal mortality—death occurring prior to, during, or within 48 hours of calving—is a recognized problem in the cattle industry.[89] In developed countries, 25% to 46% of perinatal deaths in cattle are the result of dystocia, and, in the United States, 32% of perinatal deaths are due to unknown causes. One of the main causes of dystocia is fetal-maternal size mismatch. Dystocia has a direct negative impact on calves,[89,90] dam survival and reproduction performance,[91] and milk production.[92] The authors' current research hopes to aims if similar genetic and epigenetic misregulation is the culprit of S-LOS, a previously uncharacterized syndrome in cattle, and to shed light on the contribution of S-LOS to the 25% to 46% rate of perinatal death in cattle resulting from unknown causes and dystocia.

REFERENCES

1. Lapunzina P. Risk of tumorigenesis in overgrowth syndromes: a comprehensive review. Am J Med Genet C Semin Med Genet 2005;137C(1):53–71.
2. Young LE, Sinclair KD, Wilmut I. Large offspring syndrome in cattle and sheep. Rev Reprod 1998;3(3):155–63.
3. Sinclair K, Young L, Wilmut I, et al. In-utero overgrowth in ruminants following embryo culture: lessons from mice and a warning to men. Hum Reprod 2000; 15(suppl_5):68–86.
4. Opitz JM, Weaver DW, Reynolds JF. The syndromes of Sotos and Weaver: reports and review. Am J Med Genet A 1998;79(4):294–304.
5. Elliott M, Bayly R, Cole T, et al. Clinical features and natural history of Beckwith-Wiedemann syndrome: presentation of 74 new cases. Clin Genet 1994;46(2): 168–74.
6. Wiedemann H-R, Burgio G, Aldenhoff P, et al. The proteus syndrome. Eur J Pediatr 1983;140(1):5–12.
7. Biesecker L. The challenges of Proteus syndrome: diagnosis and management. Eur J Hum Genet 2006;14(11):1151.
8. DeBaun MR, Niemitz EL, Feinberg AP. Association of in vitro fertilization with Beckwith-Wiedemann syndrome and epigenetic alterations of LIT1 and H19. Am J Hum Genet 2003;72(1):156–60.
9. Cole T, Hughes H. Sotos syndrome: a study of the diagnostic criteria and natural history. J Med Genet 1994;31(1):20–32.
10. Lazzari G, Wrenzycki C, Herrmann D, et al. Cellular and molecular deviations in bovine in vitro-produced embryos are related to the large offspring syndrome. Biol Reprod 2002;67(3):767–75.
11. Behboodi E, Anderson GB, BonDurant RH, et al. Birth of large calves that developed from in vitro-derived bovine embryos. Theriogenology 1995;44(2):227–32.
12. Hasler J, Henderson W, Hurtgen P, et al. Production, freezing and transfer of bovine IVF embryos and subsequent calving results. Theriogenology 1995; 43(1):141–52.
13. van Wagtendonk-de Leeuw AM, Mullaart E, de Roos AP, et al. Effects of different reproduction techniques: AI MOET or IVP, on health and welfare of bovine offspring. Theriogenology 2000;53(2):575–97.
14. Farin PW, Farin CE. Transfer of bovine embryos produced in vivo or in vitro: survival and fetal development. Biol Reprod 1995;52(3):676–82.
15. van Wagtendonk-de Leeuw AM, Aerts BJ, den Daas JH. Abnormal offspring following in vitro production of bovine preimplantation embryos: a field study. Theriogenology 1998;49(5):883–94.
16. Farin PW, Piedrahita JA, Farin CE. Errors in development of fetuses and placentas from in vitro-produced bovine embryos. Theriogenology 2006;65(1):178–91.
17. Walker S, Hartwich K, Seamark R. The production of unusually large offspring following embryo manipulation: concepts and challenges. Theriogenology 1996;45(1):111–20.
18. Farin P, Crosier A, Farin C. Influence of in vitro systems on embryo survival and fetal development in cattle. Theriogenology 2001;55(1):151–70.
19. Hansen PJ, Dobbs KB, Denicol AC, et al. Sex and the preimplantation embryo: implications of sexual dimorphism in the preimplantation period for maternal programming of embryonic development. Cell Tissue Res 2016;363(1):237–47.

20. Wilson J, Williams J, Bondioli K, et al. Comparison of birth weight and growth characteristics of bovine calves produced by nuclear transfer (cloning), embryo transfer and natural mating. Anim Reprod Sci 1995;38(1–2):73–83.
21. Brioude F, Kalish JM, Mussa A, et al. Expert consensus document: clinical and molecular diagnosis, screening and management of Beckwith–Wiedemann syndrome: an international consensus statement. Nat Rev Endocrinol 2018;14(4): 229–49.
22. Chen Z, Robbins KM, Wells KD, et al. Large offspring syndrome: a bovine model for the human loss-of-imprinting overgrowth syndrome Beckwith-Wiedemann. Epigenetics 2013;8(6):591–601.
23. Bair JH, Russ PD, Pretorius DH, et al. Fetal omphalocele and gastroschisis: a review of 24 cases. Am J Roentgenol 1986;147(5):1047–51.
24. Jackson OJ, Moglen L. Umbilical hernia—a retrospective study. Calif Med 1970; 113(4):8.
25. McEvoy T, Sinclair K, Broadbent P, et al. Post-natal growth and development of Simmental calves derived from in vivo or in vitro embryos. Reprod Fertil Dev 1998;10(6):459–64.
26. Sinclair K, Broadbent P, Dolman D. In vitro produced embryos as a means of achieving pregnancy and improving productivity in beef cows. Animal Science 1995;60(1):55–64.
27. Kruip TA, Den Daas J. In vitro produced and cloned embryos: effects on pregnancy, parturition and offspring. Theriogenology 1997;47(1):43–52.
28. Reichenbach H, Liebrich J, Berg U, et al. Pregnancy rates and births after unilateral or bilateral transfer of bovine embryos produced in vitro. J Reprod Fertil 1992;95(2):363–70.
29. Schmidt M, Greve T, Avery B, et al. Pregnancies, calves and calf viability after transfer of in vitro produced bovine embryos. Theriogenology 1996;46(3):527–39.
30. Barker DJ. The fetal and infant origins of disease. Eur J Clin Invest 1995;25(7): 457–63.
31. National Research Council. Methods and mechanisms for genetic manipulation of plants, animals, and microorganisms 2004.
32. Edwards R. Maturation in vitro of mouse, sheep, cow, pig, rhesus monkey and human ovarian oocytes. Nature 1965;208(5008):349.
33. Young LE, Fernandes K, McEvoy TG, et al. Epigenetic change in IGF2R is associated with fetal overgrowth after sheep embryo culture. Nat Genet 2001;27(2): 153.
34. Chen Z, Hagen DE, Elsik CG, et al. Characterization of global loss of imprinting in fetal overgrowth syndrome induced by assisted reproduction. Proc Natl Acad Sci U S A 2015;112(15):4618–23.
35. Carolan C, Lonergan P, Van Langendonckt A, et al. Factors affecting bovine embryo development in synthetic oviduct fluid following oocyte maturation and fertilization in vitro. Theriogenology 1995;43(6):1115–28.
36. Thompson J, Allen N, McGowan L, et al. Effect of delayed supplementation of fetal calf serum to culture medium on bovine embryo development in vitro and following transfer. Theriogenology 1998;49(6):1239–49.
37. Thompson JG, Gardner DK, Anne Pugh P, et al. Lamb birth weight is affected by culture system utilized during in vitro pre-elongation development of ovine embryos. Biol Reprod 1995;53(6):1385–91.
38. Gandolfi F, Moor R. Stimulation of early embryonic development in the sheep by co-culture with oviduct epithelial cells. J Reprod Fertil 1987;81(1):23–8.

39. Holm P, Walker SK, Seamark RF. Embryo viability, duration of gestation and birth weight in sheep after transfer of in vitro matured and in vitro fertilized zygotes cultured in vitro or in vivo. J Reprod Fertil 1996;107(2):175–81.
40. Maxfield E, Sinclair K, Dolman D, et al. In vitro culture of sheep embryos increases weight, primary fiber size and secondary to primary fiber ratio in fetal muscle at day 61 of gestation. Theriogenology 1997;1(47):376.
41. Mussa A, Russo S, De Crescenzo A, et al. Prevalence of Beckwith–Wiedemann syndrome in north west of Italy. Am J Med Genet A 2013;161(10):2481–6.
42. Vermeiden JP, Bernardus RE. Are imprinting disorders more prevalent after human in vitro fertilization or intracytoplasmic sperm injection? Fertil Steril 2013; 99(3):642–51.
43. Mussa A, Molinatto C, Cerrato F, et al. Assisted reproductive techniques and risk of Beckwith-Wiedemann Syndrome. Pediatrics 2017;140(1) [pii:e20164311].
44. Gicquel C, Gaston V, Mandelbaum J, et al. In vitro fertilization may increase the risk of Beckwith-Wiedemann syndrome related to the abnormal imprinting of the KCN1OT gene. Am J Hum Genet 2003;72(5):1338–41.
45. Reik W, Brown KW, Schneid H, et al. Imprinting mutations in the Beckwith—Wiedemann syndrome suggested by an altered imprinting pattern in the IGF2–H19 domain. Hum Mol Genet 1995;4(12):2379–85.
46. Henry I, Bonaiti-Pellie C, Chehensse V, et al. Uniparental paternal disomy in a genetic cancer-predisposing syndrome. Nature 1991;351(6328):665.
47. Waziri M, Patil SR, Hanson JW, et al. Abnormality of chromosome 11 in patients withfeatures of Beckwith-Wiedemann syndrome. J Pediatr 1983;102(6):873–6.
48. Schmutz SM. Deletion of chromosome 11 (p11p13) in a patient with Beckwith-Wiedemann syndrome. Clin Genet 1986;30(3):154–6.
49. Beygo J, Joksic I, Strom TM, et al. A maternal deletion upstream of the imprint control region 2 in 11p15 causes loss of methylation and familial Beckwith–Wiedemann syndrome. Eur J Hum Genet 2016;24(9):1280.
50. Okano Y, Osasa Y, Yamamoto H, et al. An infant with Beckwith-Wiedemann syndrome and chromosomal duplication 11p13→ pter.: Correlation of symptoms between 11p trisomy and Beckwith-Wiedemann syndrome. J Hum Genet 1986; 31(4):365.
51. Turleau C, de Grouchy J, Chavin-Colin F, et al. Trisomy 11p15 and Beckwith-Wiedemann syndrome. A report of two cases. Hum Genet 1984;67(2):219–21.
52. Hatada I, Ohashi H, Fukushima Y, et al. An imprinted gene p57KIP2 is mutated in Beckwith–Wiedemann syndrome. Nat Genet 1996;14(2):171.
53. Blake A, Pickford K, Greenaway S, et al. MouseBook: an integrated portal of mouse resources. Nucleic Acids Res 2010;38(Database issue):D593–9.
54. Chen Z, Hagen DE, Wang J, et al. Global assessment of imprinted gene expression in the bovine conceptus by next generation sequencing. Epigenetics 2016; 11(7):501–16.
55. Tian XC. Genomic imprinting in farm animals. Annu Rev Anim Biosci 2014;2: 23–40.
56. Morison IM, Paton CJ, Cleverley SD. The imprinted gene and parent-of-origin effect database. Nucleic Acids Res 2001;29(1):275–6.
57. Reik W, Walter J. Genomic imprinting: parental influence on the genome. Nat Rev Genet 2001;2(1):21–32.
58. Lee MP, DeBaun MR, Mitsuya K, et al. Loss of imprinting of a paternally expressed transcript, with antisense orientation to KVLQT1, occurs frequently in Beckwith–Wiedemann syndrome and is independent of insulin-like growth factor II imprinting. Proc Natl Acad Sci U S A 1999;96(9):5203–8.

59. Smilinich NJ, Day CD, Fitzpatrick GV, et al. A maternally methylated CpG island in KvLQT1 is associated with an antisense paternal transcript and loss of imprinting in Beckwith–Wiedemann syndrome. Proc Natl Acad Sci U S A 1999;96(14): 8064–9.
60. Horike S-I, Mitsuya K, Meguro M, et al. Targeted disruption of the human LIT1 locus defines a putative imprinting control element playing an essential role in Beckwith–Wiedemann syndrome. Hum Mol Genet 2000;9(14):2075–83.
61. Brioude F, Lacoste A, Netchine I, et al. Beckwith-Wiedemann syndrome: growth pattern and tumor risk according to molecular mechanism, and guidelines for tumor surveillance. Horm Res paediatrics 2013;80(6):457–65.
62. Ibrahim A, Kirby G, Hardy C, et al. Methylation analysis and diagnostics of Beckwith-Wiedemann syndrome in 1,000 subjects. Clin epigenetics 2014; 6(1):11.
63. Mussa A, Russo S, De Crescenzo A, et al. (Epi) genotype–phenotype correlations in Beckwith–Wiedemann syndrome. Eur J Hum Genet 2016;24(2):183.
64. Wrenzycki C, Herrmann D, Carnwath J, et al. Alterations in the relative abundance of gene transcripts in preimplantation bovine embryos cultured in medium supplemented with either serum or PVA. Mol Reprod Dev 1999;53(1):8–18.
65. Wrenzycki C, Herrmann D, Keskintepe L, et al. Effects of culture system and protein supplementation on mRNA expression in pre-implantation bovine embryos. Hum Reprod 2001;16(5):893–901.
66. Rizos D, Lonergan P, Boland M, et al. Analysis of differential messenger RNA expression between bovine blastocysts produced in different culture systems: implications for blastocyst quality. Biol Reprod 2002;66(3):589–95.
67. Rizos D, Gutierrez-Adan A, Perez-Garnelo S, et al. Bovine embryo culture in the presence or absence of serum: implications for blastocyst development, cryotolerance, and messenger RNA expression. Biol Reprod 2003;68(1):236–43.
68. Rizos D, Fair T, Moreira P, et al. Effect of speed of development on mRNA expression pattern in early bovine embryos cultured in vivo or in vitro. Mol Reprod Dev 2004;68(4):441–8.
69. Corcoran D, Fair T, Park S, et al. Suppressed expression of genes involved in transcription and translation in in vitro compared with in vivo cultured bovine embryos. Reproduction 2006;131(4):651–60.
70. Fair T, Carter F, Park S, et al. Global gene expression analysis during bovine oocyte in vitro maturation. Theriogenology 2007;68:S91–7.
71. Smith SL, Everts RE, Sung LY, et al. Gene expression profiling of single bovine embryos uncovers significant effects of in vitro maturation, fertilization and culture. Mol Reprod Dev 2009;76(1):38–47.
72. Driver AM, Peñagaricano F, Huang W, et al. RNA-Seq analysis uncovers transcriptomic variations between morphologically similar in vivo-and in vitro-derived bovine blastocysts. BMC Genomics 2012;13(1):118.
73. Chen Z, Hagen DE, Ji T, et al. Global misregulation of genes largely uncoupled to DNA methylome epimutations characterizes a congenital overgrowth syndrome. Sci Rep 2017;7(1):12667.
74. Blondin P, Farin PW, Crosier AE, et al. In vitro production of embryos alters levels of insulin-like growth factor-II messenger ribonucleic acid in bovine fetuses 63 days after transfer. Biol Reprod 2000;62(2):384–9.
75. Zaborski D, Grzesiak W, Szatkowska I, et al. Factors affecting dystocia in cattle. Reprod Domest Anim 2009;44(3):540–51.
76. Holland M, Odde K. Factors affecting calf birth weight: a review. Theriogenology 1992;38(5):769–98.

77. Kamien B, Ronan A, Poke G, et al. A clinical review of generalized overgrowth syndromes in the era of massively parallel sequencing. Mol Syndromol 2018; 9(2):70–82.
78. Kampmann U, Madsen LR, Skajaa GO, et al. Gestational diabetes: A clinical update. World J Diabetes 2015;6(8):1065.
79. Bianci D, Crombleholme T, Dalton M, et al. Fetology: diagnosis and management of the fetal patient. 2nd edition. McGraw-Hill Professional; 2010.
80. Foote R. Factors affecting gestation length in dairy cattle. Theriogenology 1981; 15(6):553–9.
81. Shibata S, Ishihara M. Studies on hereditary defects in Japanese native cattle. Japan. J. Zoötech. Sci 1949;19:63.
82. Graves TK, Hansel W, Krook L. Prolonged gestation in a Holstein cow: adenohypophyseal aplasia and skeletal pathology in the offspring. Cornell Vet 1991;81(3): 277–94.
83. Buczinski S, Bélanger AM, Fecteau G, et al. Prolonged gestation in two Holstein cows: transabdominal ultrasonographic findings in late pregnancy and pathologic findings in the fetuses. J Vet Med A Physiol Pathol Clin Med 2007;54(10): 624–6.
84. Cornillie P, Van den Broeck W, Simoens P. Prolonged gestation in two Belgian blue cows due to inherited adenohypophyseal hypoplasia in the fetuses. Vet Rec 2007;161:388–91.
85. Constable PD, Hinchcliff KW, Done SH, et al. Veterinary medicine : a textbook of the diseases of cattle, horses, sheep, pigs, and goats. 11th edition. Elsevier Health Sciences; 2017.
86. Roberts SJ. Veterinary obstetrics and genital diseases (theriogenology). 2nd edition. Ann Arbor (MI): Edwards Brothers Inc.; 1971.
87. Brackett BG, Bousquet D, Boice ML, et al. Normal development following in vitro fertilization in the cow. Biol Reprod 1982;27(1):147–58.
88. Hasler JF. Forty years of embryo transfer in cattle: a review focusing on the journal Theriogenology, the growth of the industry in North America, and personal reminisces. Theriogenology 2014;81(1):152–69.
89. Mee JF. Why do so many calves die on modern dairy farms and what can we do about calf welfare in the future? Animals 2013;3(4):1036–57.
90. Mee JF, Sanchez-Miguel C, Doherty M. Influence of modifiable risk factors on the incidence of stillbirth/perinatal mortality in dairy cattle. Vet J 2014;199(1):19–23.
91. Bicalho RC, Galvao KN, Cheong SH, et al. Effect of stillbirths on dam survival and reproduction performance in Holstein dairy cows. J Dairy Sci 2007;90(6): 2797–803.
92. Bicalho RC, Galvao KN, Warnick LD, et al. Stillbirth parturition reduces milk production in Holstein cows. Prev Vet Med 2008;84(1–2):112–20.

Postnatal Nutrient Repartitioning due to Adaptive Developmental Programming

Robert J. Posont, HBSC, MS, Dustin T. Yates, BS, MS, PhD*

KEYWORDS

- Developmental origins of health and disease • Fetal adaptations • Fetal stress
- Nutrient repartitioning • Thrifty phenotype

KEY POINTS

- Fetal adaptations to nutritional stress lead to intrauterine growth restriction (IUGR) and low birthweight. This occurs in all mammalian species and is a long-standing challenge to food animal production.
- IUGR fetal adaptations repartition limited nutrients to vital neural, cardiac, and endocrine tissues by restricting skeletal muscle mass and nutrient utilization.
- Nutrient-sparing adaptations aid fetal survival of IUGR conditions but become problematic after birth when nutrient supply is not limited. IUGR-born offspring have less lean muscle and increased fat deposition, which reduces feed efficiency, carcass quality, and value.
- Developmental adaptations affect fat, liver, and pancreatic β-cells, in addition to skeletal muscle. Changes include reduced tissue responsiveness to insulin, greater local inflammation, and altered β-adrenergic tone.

INTRODUCTION

The consequences of prenatal stress on lifelong metabolic function and health were first proposed by Nicholas Hales and David Barker[1,2] with the publication of their thrifty phenotype hypothesis in the early 1990s. Subsequent studies in humans and animals have further demonstrated that stress-induced adaptive fetal programming leads to tissue-specific changes in metabolic function and growth capacity.[3,4]

The authors (R.P., D.Y.) have no commercial or financial conflicts of interest to declare. This project was partially supported by the National Institute of General Medical Sciences Grant 1P20GM104320 (J. Zempleni, Director), the Nebraska Agricultural Experiment Station with funding from the Hatch Act (NEB-26-224) and Hatch Multistate Research capacity funding program (NEB-26-226, NEB-26-225) through the USDA National Institute of Food and Agriculture. Department of Animal Science, University of Nebraska–Lincoln, PO Box 830908, Lincoln, NE 68583, USA
* Corresponding author.
E-mail address: dustin.yates@unl.edu

Developmental adaptations to the intrauterine nutrient restriction that accompanies most maternofetal stressors target regulatory pathways for nutrient utilization in nonessential tissues such as skeletal muscle.[4–6] This aids intrauterine survival by reappropriating nutrients to support neural, cardiac, and endocrine tissue function but reduces metabolic efficiency and growth capacity in offspring. Stress-induced fetal adaptations are typically characterized by intrauterine growth restriction (IUGR) during late gestation and by low birthweight.[7,8] Poor postnatal growth and metabolic inefficiency associated with low birthweight can reduce value in livestock.[4,8] Experimental models of IUGR livestock show how maternofetal stress from environmental, nutritional, or health conditions lead to fetal metabolic adaptations[5,9,10]; however, few studies have followed IUGR-born livestock after birth. Even less is known about how adaptive changes alter nutrient utilization in these offspring. This article summarizes the current literature that assesses nutrient partitioning in IUGR-born animals and describes the key adaptive mechanisms underlying developmental changes that reduce muscle growth and impair metabolism.

THE INTRAUTERINE GROWTH RESTRICTION PHENOTYPE
Intrauterine Growth Restriction Is a Product of Developmental Adaptations

Studies in IUGR fetal sheep and other animals show that asymmetric fetal growth restriction is a consequence of nutrient-sparing developmental adaptations.[5,11] These adaptations most commonly result from placental insufficiency produced by sustained maternal stress during midgestation.[11,12] Placental insufficiency can result from several environmental challenges, including heat stress, nutrient restriction, and illness, but produces consistent developmental outcomes in the fetus.[12,13] Regardless of the maternal or placental insult, placental insufficiency induces changes in metabolic tissues such as skeletal muscle, pancreas, liver, and adipose tissues[14–16] (**Table 1**).

Table 1
Low birthweight animals exhibit multitissue pathologic conditions that alter nutrient partitioning and contribute to inefficient growth and metabolism

Low Birthweight Pathologic Conditions	Potential Underlying Mechanism
Skeletal Muscle	
↓ Myoblast Function	↓ β2-adrenergic to β1-adrenergic activity
↓ Hypertrophic Growth	↑ Inflammatory sensitivity or responsiveness
↓ Glucose Oxidation	Δ Fiber type ratios
↓ Protein Accretion	
Adipose Tissue	
↑ Visceral Fat Deposition	↑ Macrophage infiltration
↑ Adipocyte Proliferation	↑ PPARγ
	↑ Lipogenic proteins
	↑ Nutrient delivery
Liver	
↓ Mass	↓ Nutrient-sensing proteins (AMPK, mTOR, sirtuin 1)
↑ Triglyceride Accumulation	↑ Hepatic inflammation
? Gluconeogenesis	↓ Fatty acid oxidation
Pancreatic β-cells	
↓ Glucose-Stimulated Insulin Secretion	Δ Adrenergic regulation
↓ Insulin Production	↓ Glucose oxidation

↑, increase; ↓, decrease; ?, unknown.

Together, these collective adaptive responses alter systemic nutrient repartitioning by reducing substrate utilization by nonvisceral soft tissues in favor of critical brain, heart, lungs, and endocrine tissues.[13,17] Restriction of skeletal muscle growth, insulin sensitivity, and pancreatic function are chief among these fetal adaptations.[3,11,14–16]

Intrauterine Growth Restriction Adaptations Persist in Offspring

Thrifty metabolic adaptations that develop during gestation persist after birth despite alleviation of prenatal stressors.[2,18] The first evidence that prenatal stress is associated with postnatal metabolic dysfunction arose from Barker's epidemiologic studies of socioeconomic classes in the United Kingdom.[1,2] In poorer industrial populations, high rates of low birthweight infants correlated with greater incidence of hypertension, obesity, type 2 diabetes, and glucose intolerance in adulthood.[1,2] Low birthweight individuals also exhibit lifelong reductions in lean mass and increased fat deposition.[19–21] These results have since been corroborated in other human populations.[22,23] Moreover, low birthweight livestock exhibit similar changes in body composition and metabolic function[18,24,25] (**Fig. 1**). Recent research by the authors' laboratory and others has focused on understanding the molecular mechanisms that link developmental adaptations in utero with lifelong changes in metabolic function, nutrient utilization, and growth capacity.

POSTNATAL GROWTH CHARACTERISTICS IN INTRAUTERINE GROWTH RESTRICTION–BORN LIVESTOCK
Low Birthweight Animals Exhibit Altered Body Composition

Similar to low birthweight children,[26] low birthweight animals demonstrate accelerated neonatal catch-up growth that is driven by increased fat deposition rather than muscle growth.[18,27] In fact, persistence of poor muscle growth leads to a reduction in carcass yield, smaller high-value cuts from the loin and upper hindlimb, and increased fat thickness in both cattle and sheep.[18,28] Reduced muscle growth and increased adiposity seem to occur via independent mechanisms and it is worth noting that fat deposits are actually reduced in the IUGR fetus due to greater mobilization.[29] Greater adiposity in offspring seems to be secondary to impaired muscle growth because a smaller proportion of dietary nutrients are used for muscle growth and thus more nutrients are stored as fat.[18,30] Conversely, studies by the authors' laboratory and others show that impaired skeletal muscle growth is the product of intrinsic myoblast dysfunction.[12,14,31,32]

Skeletal Muscle Growth Is Disproportionally Reduced

Reduced lean mass and muscle size in low birthweight livestock at harvest[28,33–36] is the result of impaired hypertrophic muscle growth. In IUGR fetal sheep, cross-sectional areas of hindlimb muscle fibers reduced by as much as 50% but no reduction in fiber numbers were observed.[14,31] Muscle fibers remained smaller in IUGR-born lambs at 1 month of age, or approximately 20 kg bodyweight.[28,37] Myoblast function is the rate-limiting step in hypertrophic muscle growth,[38] and impaired skeletal muscle growth in IUGR fetal and neonatal sheep coincided with intrinsic deficits in myoblast proliferative and differentiation capacities.[31,32,37,39] Skeletal muscle is the greatest utilizer of glucose in the body,[40,41] and utilization per gram of muscle is not reduced in the IUGR fetus or lamb.[10,11,42] Thus, restricting skeletal muscle mass is a key mechanism for repartitioning the limited glucose supply in the IUGR fetus from muscle to vital tissue function and development. However, persistent deficits in muscle growth capacity in IUGR-born livestock reduce their value in meat production.[4]

Nutrient Partitioning in Low Birthweight Livestock

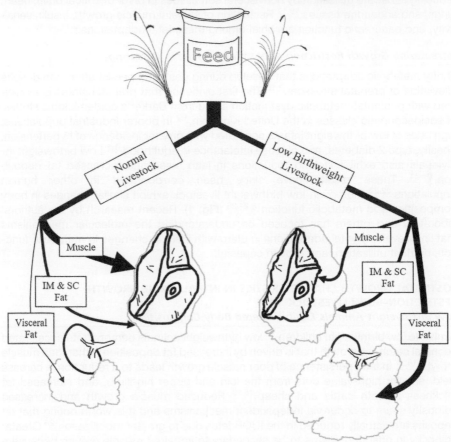

Fig. 1. Stress-induced fetal adaptations cause low birthweight livestock to reappropriate dietary nutrients. Less nutrients are used for skeletal muscle growth and more are redirected to visceral fat deposits and, to a lesser extent, intramuscular (IM) and subcutaneous (SC) fat deposits.

Skeletal Muscle Protein Accretion Is Reduced

Similar to glucose, skeletal muscle in low birthweight livestock use less protein during early growth.[28] Recent studies by Laura Brown's laboratory help point out several key mechanisms for adaptive changes in muscle protein utilization.[43,44] As IUGR fetuses approach term, their rates of skeletal muscle protein breakdown remain comparable to uncompromised fetuses.[43] However, protein synthesis and accretion rates in IUGR skeletal muscle drop by as much as 50%, which is similar to reduction in amino acid uptake and utilization.[43] Moreover, the effects of IUGR on circulating amino acid concentrations vary widely among individual amino acids.[43,44] For example, tyrosine, arginine, and isoleucine concentrations were reduced in IUGR fetal blood; however, taurine, glycine, and alanine concentrations were increased.[43] Increasing amino acid supply via direct fetal infusion did not increase protein accretion or synthesis rates, muscle size, or fetal mass but increased amino acid oxidation rates.[44] Thus, reduced protein uptake and accretion by IUGR skeletal muscle does not seem to be the direct result of reduced fetal protein availability. Rather, it may be a product of β-adrenergic adaptations due to chronic hypercatecholaminemia because hypercatecholaminemia was not mitigated by amino acid infusion in this study. β2-adrenergic stimulation increases protein synthesis and cycling[45] but gene expression for the β2-adrenergic receptor is reduced in IUGR skeletal muscle.[4] When hypercatecholaminemia was mitigated by adrenal demedullation in IUGR fetal sheep, fetal mass was increased by 50% to 60%.[46,47] Diminished blood flow, reduced oxygen utilization, and hypoinsulinemia may also contribute to reduced protein accretion in IUGR muscle.[43,48]

TISSUE-SPECIFIC METABOLIC CHANGES IN INTRAUTERINE GROWTH RESTRICTION LIVESTOCK

Skeletal Muscle Glucose Metabolism Is Altered

In humans, skeletal muscle from IUGR-born individuals show evidence of impaired insulin responsiveness and reduced glucose oxidative metabolism.[22,23,49–51] Studies in IUGR fetal sheep show that reduced whole-body glucose oxidation rates are present near term and occur despite normal rates of glucose uptake and utilization.[10,11] It was shown that reduced glucose oxidation is muscle-specific in the IUGR fetal sheep and neonatal lamb.[4,52,53] In concert with reduced glucose oxidation, IUGR skeletal muscle increases lactate production,[9,10,41] which, unlike glucose, can be secreted from skeletal muscle. Lactate can then be used by the liver for glucose production or by cardiac tissue for energy.[11,54,55] The shift in IUGR skeletal muscle glucose metabolism coincides with a reduction in the proportion of oxidative muscle fibers relative to glycolytic fibers.[14] The authors are not aware of any studies measuring muscle fiber types in low birthweight offspring of ruminant livestock; however, reductions in oxidative-to-glycolytic muscle fiber types have been observed in IUGR-born humans[56] and mice.[57]

Like reduced muscle growth, the metabolic shift in IUGR skeletal muscle seems to be at least partially due to changes in adrenergic activity. Studies by the authors' laboratory and others have shown that skeletal muscle insulin action and glucose oxidation are stimulated by β2-adrenergic activity but reduced by β1-adrenergic activity.[58–60] Fetal hypoxemia increases circulating catecholamine levels[61] and chronic adrenergic exposure during late gestation reduces β2-adrenergic to β1-adrenergic receptor gene expression in IUGR skeletal muscle.[4] It is worth noting that slow oxidative muscle fibers express more β-adrenergic receptors than fast glycolytic fibers[62,63] and thus may be affected by chronic hypercatecholaminemia to a greater extent.

Fat Deposition Is Increased

Adaptive changes in IUGR skeletal muscle nutrient utilization cause a greater proportion of dietary nutrients to be deposited into central fat stores.[18,26,35] In addition, IUGR fetal adipocytes undergo developmental adaptations that increase their ability to proliferate and expand in size, which increases their ability to store more fat.[64] IUGR-born male rats indicate that a possible adaptive mechanism is the increased activity of peroxisome proliferator-activated receptor (PPAR) gamma, which is a primary regulator of adipogenesis and lipogenesis.[16] Other studies have implicated greater expression of the lipogenic proteins, acetyl-CoA carboxylase-α, fatty acid synthase, and ATP-binding cassette transporter 1.[65,66]

Adipose tissue plays an indirect role in systemic metabolic regulation related to its effects on endocrine and immune function, and greater fat mass in IUGR-born animals disrupts these functions.[67] Immunomodulatory disruptions in IUGR-born ruminants precede obesity and are attributable to increased infiltration of macrophages into visceral and subcutaneous fat depots, creating tissue inflammation that further contributes to insulin resistance, metabolic dysfunction, and poor growth.[67,68] Hyperlipidemia also increases systemic inflammation in humans,[69] although the authors are not aware of any similar studies in ruminant livestock. This occurs via activation of toll-like receptor 4 (TLR4) by free fatty acids, which in turn upregulates inflammatory pathways that impair insulin signaling and induce metabolic dysfunction.[69]

Changes in Hepatic Function Contribute to Metabolic Dysfunction

Lipid homeostasis is regulated in large part by liver function, and adaptations in hepatic development contribute to metabolic dysfunction in IUGR offspring.[70–72] In sheep, IUGR liver mass is reduced in the near-term fetus and in offspring.[71,73] Hepatic expression of gluconeogenic enzymes, including phosphoenolpyruvate carboxykinase (PEPCK) and glucose 6-phosphatase (G6P), are increased in response to chronic hypoglycemia near term.[11,71] However, the impact on postnatal gluconeogenesis is less clear because gluconeogenic enzymes remain elevated into adulthood in IUGR-born rats[74,75] but are normal or even reduced in IUGR-born lambs.[76,77] Conversely, hepatic glycogen content is normal in IUGR fetal sheep[11,71] but reduced at 1 month of age.[73]

Hepatic adaptations in the IUGR fetus diminish activation of nutrient-sensing proteins, including AMPK, mTOR, and sirtuin 1.[71] This adaptation likely spares fetal hepatocytes from apoptosis but also contributes to hepatic inflammation, dyslipidemia, and reduced insulin responsiveness in offspring.[70,71,78] These pathologic conditions are likely mediated at least in part by persistent reductions in the expression of PPARα and PPARγ.[70] Reduced lipogenesis in concert with dyslipidemia and reduced fatty acid oxidation enhance inflammatory responses in the liver and increase the synthesis of triglycerides,[70] further contributing to systemic insulin desensitization.

β-Cell Dysfunction Impairs Insulin Secretion

Insulin secretion from pancreatic β-cells is the primary regulator of glucose uptake and metabolism, and contributes to anabolic processes and muscle growth.[15,79] β-cell dysfunction is a chief factor in increased risk for metabolic dysfunction IUGR offspring.[15] In low birthweight lambs, insulin stimulus-secretion coupling is enhanced at 1 week[42] and 2 months of age[80] due to residual compensation in sensitivity to glucose that develops in utero.[80–82] Compensatory increases are transient, however, and adaptive impairment of glucose-stimulated insulin secretion is apparent by 8 months of age[80] (Fig. 2). The severity of β-cell dysfunction is typically proportional to the severity of placental insufficiency and is, at least in part, associated with impaired islet development.[15,83] IUGR fetal sheep exhibit reduced β-cell mass and intracellular insulin concentrations near term, despite minimal effects on other endocrine cell types within the islets.[15,83,84] This seems to be the product of changes in adrenergic regulation due to chronic fetal hypercatecholaminemia, which altered catecholamine-responsive genes associated with both cellular development and function.[85] In addition, islets isolated from these fetuses impaired glucose oxidation capacity,[83,84] which is a key step in secretion-stimulus coupling. Developmental adaptations in IUGR fetal islets seem to be the result of chronic adrenergic exposure because 7-day norepinephrine infusion into otherwise uncompromised fetal sheep produced similar effects.[86,87]

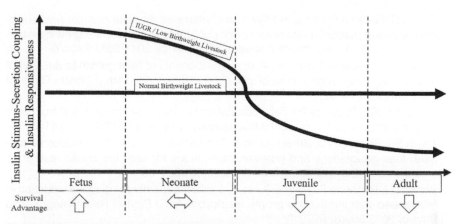

Fig. 2. Stress-induced fetal adaptations impair tissue responsiveness to insulin. In prenatal and early postnatal stages, impaired insulin action is masked by transient increases in insulin sensitivity, which benefits IUGR fetal survival.

SUMMARY

Stress-induced adaptive fetal programming leads to IUGR and low birthweight. Low birthweight livestock are characterized by changes in nutrient partitioning, tissue-specific metabolic function, growth, and body composition. Studies in cattle and sheep show that these adaptations result in poor growth efficiency and carcass value. Skeletal muscle nutrient utilization seems to be disproportionately targeted by fetal adaptations to stress because glucose oxidation and protein accretion are impaired. These changes coincide with reductions in slow oxidative fiber proportions, insulin responsiveness, hypertrophic growth, and β2-adrenergic stimulation. In low birth-weight offspring, adaptations reduce nutrient utilization for muscle growth. Instead, a greater amount of dietary nutrients are stored as visceral fat. Adaptive changes in functional development of adipocytes, liver tissues, and pancreatic β-cells further contribute to metabolic inefficiency and body composition changes. Poor muscle growth together with greater fat deposition leads to less efficient feed conversion, lower yields, smaller high-value cuts, and reduced value in low birthweight livestock.

REFERENCES

1. Hales C, Barker D, Clark P, et al. Fetal and infant growth and impaired glucose tolerance at age 64. BMJ 1991;303(6809):1019–22.

2. Hales CN, Barker DJ. Type 2 (non-insulin-dependent) diabetes mellitus: the thrifty phenotype hypothesis. Diabetologia 1992;35(7):595–601.

3. Funston RN, Summers AF. Effect of prenatal programming on heifer development. Vet Clin North Am Food Anim Pract 2013;29(3):517–36.

4. Yates DT, Petersen JL, Schmidt TB, et al. ASAS-SSR Triennnial Reproduction Symposium: looking back and moving forward-how reproductive physiology has evolved: fetal origins of impaired muscle growth and metabolic dysfunction: lessons from the heat-stressed pregnant ewe. J Anim Sci 2018;96(7):2987–3002.

5. Yates DT, Macko AR, Nearing M, et al. Developmental programming in response to intrauterine growth restriction impairs myoblast function and skeletal muscle metabolism. J Pregnancy 2012;2012:631038.

6. Yates DT, Green AS, Limesand SW. Catecholamines mediate multiple fetal adaptations during placental insufficiency that contribute to intrauterine growth restriction: lessons from hyperthermic sheep. J Pregnancy 2011;2011:740408.

7. Galan HL, Hussey MJ, Barbera A, et al. Relationship of fetal growth to duration of heat stress in an ovine model of placental insufficiency. Am J Obstet Gynecol 1999;180(5):1278–82.

8. Limesand SW, Rozance PJ. Fetal adaptations in insulin secretion result from high catecholamines during placental insufficiency. J Physiol 2017;595(15):5103–13.

9. Thorn SR, Rozance PJ, Brown LD, et al. The intrauterine growth restriction phenotype: fetal adaptations and potential implications for later life insulin resistance and diabetes. Semin Reprod Med 2011;29(03):225–36.

10. Brown LD, Rozance PJ, Bruce JL, et al. Limited capacity for glucose oxidation in fetal sheep with intrauterine growth restriction. Am J Physiol Regul Integr Comp Physiol 2015;309(8):R920–8.

11. Limesand SW, Rozance PJ, Smith D, et al. Increased insulin sensitivity and maintenance of glucose utilization rates in fetal sheep with placental insufficiency and intrauterine growth restriction. Am J Physiol Endocrinol Metab 2007;293(6): E1716–25.

12. Soto SM, Blake AC, Wesolowski SR, et al. Myoblast replication is reduced in the IUGR fetus despite maintained proliferative capacity in vitro. J Endocrinol 2017; 232(3):475–91.

13. Morrison JL. Sheep models of intrauterine growth restriction: fetal adaptations and consequences. Clin Exp Pharmacol Physiol 2008;35(7):730–43.

14. Yates DT, Cadaret CN, Beede KA, et al. Intrauterine growth-restricted sheep fetuses exhibit smaller hindlimb muscle fibers and lower proportions of insulin-sensitive Type I fibers near term. Am J Physiol Regul Integr Comp Physiol 2016;310(11):R1020–9.

15. Boehmer BH, Limesand SW, Rozance PJ. The impact of IUGR on pancreatic islet development and beta-cell function. J Endocrinol 2017;235(2):R63–76.

16. Joss-Moore LA, Wang Y, Campbell MS, et al. Uteroplacental insufficiency increases visceral adiposity and visceral adipose PPARgamma2 expression in male rat offspring prior to the onset of obesity. Early Hum Dev 2010;86(3):179–85.

17. Rosenberg A. The IUGR newborn. Paper presented at: Seminars in perinatology. 2008.

18. De Blasio MJ, Gatford KL, Robinson JS, et al. Placental restriction of fetal growth reduces size at birth and alters postnatal growth, feeding activity, and adiposity in the young lamb. Am J Physiol Regul Integr Comp Physiol 2007;292(2):R875–86.

19. Hediger ML, Overpeck MD, Kuczmarski RJ, et al. Muscularity and fatness of infants and young children born small- or large-for-gestational-age. Pediatrics 1998;102(5):E60.

20. Kensara OA, Wootton SA, Phillips DI, et al. Fetal programming of body composition: relation between birth weight and body composition measured with dual-energy X-ray absorptiometry and anthropometric methods in older Englishmen. Am J Clin Nutr 2005;82(5):980–7.

21. Yliharsila H, Kajantie E, Osmond C, et al. Birth size, adult body composition and muscle strength in later life. Int J Obes 2007;31(9):1392–9.

22. Flanagan DE, Moore VM, Godsland IF, et al. Fetal growth and the physiological control of glucose tolerance in adults: a minimal model analysis. Am J Physiol Endocrinol Metab 2000;278(4):E700–6.

23. Ong KK, Ahmed ML, Emmett PM, et al. Association between postnatal catch-up growth and obesity in childhood: prospective cohort study. BMJ 2000;320(7240): 967–71.

24. Gondret F, Lefaucheur L, Louveau I, et al. Influence of piglet birth weight on post-natal growth performance, tissue lipogenic capacity and muscle histological traits at market weight. Livest Prod Sci 2005;93(2):137–46.

25. De Blasio MJ, Gatford KL, McMillen IC, et al. Placental restriction of fetal growth increases insulin action, growth, and adiposity in the young lamb. Endocrinology 2007;148(3):1350–8.

26. Zarrati M, Shidfar F, Razmpoosh E, et al. Does low birth weight predict hypertension and obesity in schoolchildren? Ann Nutr Metab 2013;63(1–2):69–76.

27. Madsen JG, Bee G. Compensatory growth feeding strategy does not overcome negative effects on growth and carcass composition of low birth weight pigs. Animal 2015;9(3):427–36.

28. Greenwood PL, Hunt AS, Hermanson JW, et al. Effects of birth weight and post-natal nutrition on neonatal sheep: II. Skeletal muscle growth and development. J Anim Sci 2000;78(1):50–61.

29. Gondret F, Père M-C, Tacher S, et al. Spontaneous intra-uterine growth restriction modulates the endocrine status and the developmental expression of genes in porcine fetal and neonatal adipose tissue. Gen Comp Endocrinol 2013;194: 208–16.

30. Liu H, Schultz CG, De Blasio MJ, et al. Effect of placental restriction and neonatal exendin-4 treatment on postnatal growth, adult body composition, and in vivo glucose metabolism in the sheep. Am J Physiol Endocrinol Metab 2015;309(6): E589–600.

31. Yates DT, Clarke DS, Macko AR, et al. Myoblasts from intrauterine growth-restricted sheep fetuses exhibit intrinsic deficiencies in proliferation that contribute to smaller semitendinosus myofibres. J Physiol 2014;592(Pt 14): 3113–25.

32. Posont R, Beede K, Limesand S, et al. Changes in myoblast responsiveness to TNFa and IL-6 contribute to decreased skeletal muscle mass in intrauterine growth restricted fetal sheep. Translational Animal Science 2018;2(Suppl1): S44–7.

33. Hegarty PV, Allen CE. Effect of pre-natal runting on the post-natal development of skeletal muscles in swine and rats. J Anim Sci 1978;46(6):1634–40.

34. Powell SE, Aberle ED. Skeletal muscle and adipose tissue cellularity in runt and normal birth weight swine. J Anim Sci 1981;52(4):748–56.

35. Greenwood PL, Cafe LM. Prenatal and pre-weaning growth and nutrition of cattle: long-term consequences for beef production. Animal 2007;1(9):1283–96.

36. Greenwood PL, Hunt AS, Hermanson JW, et al. Effects of birth weight and post-natal nutrition on neonatal sheep: I. Body growth and composition, and some aspects of energetic efficiency. J Anim Sci 1998;76(9):2354–67.

37. Camacho LE, Yates DT, Davenport HM, et al. Decreased satellite cell proliferation rates contribute to small fibers in the semitendinosus muscle of intrauterine growth restricted lambs. Reprod Sci 2016;23(Supplement 1):316A.

38. Allen DL, Roy RR, Edgerton VR. Myonuclear domains in muscle adaptation and disease. Muscle Nerve 1999;22(10):1350–60.

39. Greenwood PL, Slepetis RM, Bell AW, et al. Intrauterine growth retardation is associated with reduced cell cycle activity, but not myofibre number, in ovine fetal muscle. Reprod Fertil Dev 1999;11(5):281–91.

40. DeFronzo RA, Jacot E, Jequier E, et al. The effect of insulin on the disposal of intravenous glucose. Results from indirect calorimetry and hepatic and femoral venous catheterization. Diabetes 1981;30(12):1000–7.

41. Brown LD. Endocrine regulation of fetal skeletal muscle growth: impact on future metabolic health. J Endocrinol 2014;221(2):R13–29.

42. Camacho LE, Chen X, Hay WW Jr, et al. Enhanced insulin secretion and insulin sensitivity in young lambs with placental insufficiency-induced intrauterine growth restriction. Am J Physiol Regul Integr Comp Physiol 2017;313(2):R101–9.

43. Rozance PJ, Zastoupil L, Wesolowski SR, et al. Skeletal muscle protein accretion rates and hindlimb growth are reduced in late gestation intrauterine growth-restricted fetal sheep. J Physiol 2018;596(1):67–82.

44. Wai SG, Rozance PJ, Wesolowski SR, et al. Prolonged amino acid infusion into intrauterine growth restricted fetal sheep increases leucine oxidation rates. Am J Physiol Endocrinol Metab 2018;315(6):E1143–53.

45. Hostrup M, Reitelseder S, Jessen S, et al. Beta2-adrenoceptor agonist salbutamol increases protein turnover rates and alters signalling in skeletal muscle after resistance exercise in young men. J Physiol 2018;596(17):4121–39.

46. Macko AR, Yates DT, Chen X, et al. Adrenal demedullation and oxygen supplementation independently increase glucose-stimulated insulin concentrations in fetal sheep with intrauterine growth restriction. Endocrinology 2016;157(5):2104–15.

47. Davis MA, Macko AR, Steyn LV, et al. Fetal adrenal demedullation lowers circulating norepinephrine and attenuates growth restriction but not reduction of endocrine cell mass in an ovine model of intrauterine growth restriction. Nutrients 2015;7(1):500–16.

48. Limesand SW, Rozance PJ, Brown LD, et al. Effects of chronic hypoglycemia and euglycemic correction on lysine metabolism in fetal sheep. Am J Physiol Endocrinol Metab 2009;296(4):E879–87.

49. Mericq V, Ong KK, Bazaes R, et al. Longitudinal changes in insulin sensitivity and secretion from birth to age three years in small- and appropriate-for-gestational-age children. Diabetologia 2005;48(12):2609–14.

50. Jornayvaz FR, Selz R, Tappy L, et al. Metabolism of oral glucose in children born small for gestational age: evidence for an impaired whole body glucose oxidation. Metabolism 2004;53(7):847–51.

51. Ozanne S, Jensen C, Tingey K, et al. Low birthweight is associated with specific changes in muscle insulin-signalling protein expression. Diabetologia 2005;48(3):547–52.

52. Cadaret C, Merrick E, Barnes T, et al. Sustained maternal inflammation during the early third trimester yields fetal adaptations that impair subsequent skeletal muscle growth and glucose metabolism in sheep. Translational Animal Science 2018;2(Suppl1):S14–8.

53. Merrick EM, Cadaret CN, Barnes TL, et al. Metabolic regulation by stress systems in bovine myoblasts and ovine fetal skeletal muscle. Proc West Sect Am Soc Anim Sci 2017;68:87–91.

54. Barry JS, Davidsen ML, Limesand SW, et al. Developmental changes in ovine myocardial glucose transporters and insulin signaling following hyperthermia-induced intrauterine fetal growth restriction. Exp Biol Med (Maywood) 2006;231(5):566–75.

55. Thorn SR, Brown LD, Rozance PJ, et al. Increased hepatic glucose production in fetal sheep with intrauterine growth restriction is not suppressed by insulin. Diabetes 2013;62(1):65–73.

56. Jensen CB, Storgaard H, Madsbad S, et al. Altered skeletal muscle fiber composition and size precede whole-body insulin resistance in young men with low birth weight. J Clin Endocrinol Metab 2007;92(4):1530–4.

57. Beauchamp B, Ghosh S, Dysart MW, et al. Low birth weight is associated with adiposity, impaired skeletal muscle energetics and weight loss resistance in mice. Int J Obes (Lond) 2015;39(4):702–11.

58. Cadaret CN, Beede KA, Riley HE, et al. Acute exposure of primary rat soleus muscle to zilpaterol HCl (beta2 adrenergic agonist), TNFalpha, or IL-6 in culture increases glucose oxidation rates independent of the impact on insulin signaling or glucose uptake. Cytokine 2017;96:107–13.

59. Barnes T, Kubik R, Cadaret C, et al. Identifying hyperthermia in heat-stressed lambs and its effects on β agonist–stimulated glucose oxidation in muscle. Proc West Sect Am Soc Anim Sci 2017;68:106–10.

60. Hoeks J, van Baak MA, Hesselink MKC, et al. Effect of β1- and β2-adrenergic stimulation on energy expenditure, substrate oxidation, and UCP3 expression in humans. Am J Physiol Endocrinol Metab 2003;285(4):E775–82.

61. Yates DT, Macko AR, Chen X, et al. Hypoxaemia-induced catecholamine secretion from adrenal chromaffin cells inhibits glucose-stimulated hyperinsulinaemia in fetal sheep. J Physiol 2012;590(21):5439–47.

62. Williams RS, Caron MG, Daniel K. Skeletal muscle beta-adrenergic receptors: variations due to fiber type and training. Am J Physiol 1984;246(2 Pt 1):E160–7.

63. Martin W, Murphree S, Saffitz J. Beta-adrenergic receptor distribution among muscle fiber types and resistance arterioles of white, red, and intermediate skeletal muscle. Circ Res 1989;64(6):1096–105.

64. Desai M, Ross MG. Fetal programming of adipose tissue: effects of intrauterine growth restriction and maternal obesity/high-fat diet. Semin Reprod Med 2011; 29(3):237–45.

65. Yee JK, Han G, Vega J, et al. Fatty acid de novo synthesis in adult intrauterine growth-restricted offspring, and adult male response to a high fat diet. Lipids 2016;51(12):1339–51.

66. Zinkhan EK, Yu B, Callaway CW, et al. Intrauterine growth restriction combined with a maternal high-fat diet increased adiposity and serum corticosterone levels in adult rat offspring. J Dev Orig Health Dis 2018;9(3):315–28.

67. Ampem G, Azegrouz H, Bacsadi A, et al. Adipose tissue macrophages in nonrodent mammals: a comparative study. Cell Tissue Res 2016;363(2):461–78.

68. Veiga-Lopez A, Moeller J, Sreedharan R, et al. Developmental programming: interaction between prenatal BPA exposure and postnatal adiposity on metabolic variables in female sheep. Am J Physiol Endocrinol Metab 2016;310(3):E238–47.

69. Reyna SM, Ghosh S, Tantiwong P, et al. Elevated toll-like receptor 4 expression and signaling in muscle from insulin-resistant subjects. Diabetes 2008;57(10): 2595–602.

70. Alisi A, Panera N, Agostoni C, et al. Intrauterine growth retardation and nonalcoholic Fatty liver disease in children. Int J Endocrinol 2011;2011:269853.

71. Thorn SR, Regnault TR, Brown LD, et al. Intrauterine growth restriction increases fetal hepatic gluconeogenic capacity and reduces messenger ribonucleic acid translation initiation and nutrient sensing in fetal liver and skeletal muscle. Endocrinology 2009;150(7):3021–30.

72. Roberts A, Nava S, Bocconi L, et al. Liver function tests and glucose and lipid metabolism in growth-restricted fetuses. Obstet Gynecol 1999;94(2):290–4.

73. Hyatt MA, Butt EA, Budge H, et al. Effects of maternal cold exposure and nutrient restriction on the ghrelin receptor, the GH-IGF axis, and metabolic regulation in the postnatal ovine liver. Reproduction 2008;135(5):723–32.

74. Luo K, Chen P, Xie Z, et al. Effect of intrauterine growth retardation on gluconeogenic enzymes in rat liver. Zhong Nan Da Xue Xue Bao Yi Xue Ban 2014;39(4): 395–400.

75. Lane RH, MacLennan NK, Hsu JL, et al. Increased hepatic peroxisome proliferator-activated receptor-gamma coactivator-1 gene expression in a rat model of intrauterine growth retardation and subsequent insulin resistance. Endocrinology 2002;143(7):2486–90.

76. Rattanatray L, Muhlhausler BS, Nicholas LM, et al. Impact of maternal overnutrition on gluconeogenic factors and methylation of the phosphoenolpyruvate carboxykinase promoter in the fetal and postnatal liver. Pediatr Res 2014;75(1–1): 14–21.

77. Nicholas LM, Rattanatray L, MacLaughlin SM, et al. Differential effects of maternal obesity and weight loss in the periconceptional period on the epigenetic regulation of hepatic insulin-signaling pathways in the offspring. FASEB J 2013;27(9): 3786–96.

78. Magee TR, Han G, Cherian B, et al. Down-regulation of transcription factor peroxisome proliferator-activated receptor in programmed hepatic lipid dysregulation and inflammation in intrauterine growth-restricted offspring. Am J Obstet Gynecol 2008;199(3):271.e1-5.

79. Fu Z, Gilbert ER, Liu D. Regulation of insulin synthesis and secretion and pancreatic Beta-cell dysfunction in diabetes. Curr Diabetes Rev 2013;9(1):25–53.

80. Ford SP, Hess BW, Schwope MM, et al. Maternal undernutrition during early to mid-gestation in the ewe results in altered growth, adiposity, and glucose tolerance in male offspring. J Anim Sci 2007;85(5):1285–94.

81. Macko AR, Yates DT, Chen X, et al. Elevated plasma norepinephrine inhibits insulin secretion, but adrenergic blockade reveals enhanced β-cell responsiveness in an ovine model of placental insufficiency at 0.7 of gestation. J Dev Orig Health Dis 2013;4(05):402–10.

82. Leos RA, Anderson MJ, Chen X, et al. Chronic exposure to elevated norepinephrine suppresses insulin secretion in fetal sheep with placental insufficiency and intrauterine growth restriction. Am J Physiol Endocrinol Metab 2010;298(4): E770–8.

83. Limesand SW, Rozance PJ, Macko AR, et al. Reductions in insulin concentrations and beta-cell mass precede growth restriction in sheep fetuses with placental insufficiency. Am J Physiol Endocrinol Metab 2013;304(5):E516–23.

84. Limesand SW, Rozance PJ, Zerbe GO, et al. Attenuated insulin release and storage in fetal sheep pancreatic islets with intrauterine growth restriction. Endocrinology 2006;147(3):1488–97.

85. Kelly AC, Bidwell CA, Chen X, et al. Chronic adrenergic signaling causes abnormal RNA expression of proliferative genes in fetal sheep islets. Endocrinology 2018;159(10):3565–78.

86. Chen X, Green AS, Macko AR, et al. Enhanced insulin secretion responsiveness and islet adrenergic desensitization after chronic norepinephrine suppression is discontinued in fetal sheep. Am J Physiol Endocrinol Metab 2014;306(1):E58–64.

87. Chen X, Kelly AC, Yates DT, et al. Islet adaptations in fetal sheep persist following chronic exposure to high norepinephrine. J Endocrinol 2017;232(2):285–95.

The Effects of Developmental Programming upon Neonatal Mortality

V.E.A. Perry, PhD[a],*, K.J. Copping, PhD[a], G. Miguel-Pacheco, DVM, MSc, PhD[b],
J. Hernandez- Medrano, DVM, MSc, PhD[c]

KEYWORDS

- Fetal programming • Calf • Neonate • Neonatal mortality

KEY POINTS

- The maternal environment (nutrition and physiologic status) can influence neonatal mortality and morbidity.
- The effects of gestational nutrition on birth weight, dystocia, and calf survival vary with the timing and duration of dietary interventions and the sex of the offspring.
- The ability to thermoregulate, stand, suckle, and ingest sufficient quantities of colostrum is critical to neonate survival and may be altered by in utero environment.
- The quantity of colostral immunoglobulins ingested by the neonate may be affected by prenatal ambient temperature and gestational diet.
- Gestational dietary restriction may alter thyroid function and diminish brown adipose tissue capacity concomitantly effecting lymphoid atrophy and neonatal immune function.

INTRODUCTION

The greatest loss in ruminant production systems occurs during the neonatal period, that is, between birth and 28 days of life. In extensive production systems, neonatal losses are reportedly between 10% and 30% and 6% and 16% for lambs and calves,

Funding: We are grateful to the UK Agriculture and Horticulture Development Board (AHDB) funding grant entitled "Increasing lifetime productivity of the heifer" # 61100019 to VEAP and the AHDB Research Fellowship to JHM for the completion of this work. We are also grateful to the Australian Research Council (ARC) for linkage grants LP0669781 and LP110100649 awarded to VEAP enabling the completion of this work.
[a] Robinson Institute, University of Adelaide, Frome Road, South Australia 5001, Australia; [b] School of Veterinary and Medical Science, University of Nottingham, Sutton Bonington Campus, Loughborough, Leicestershire, LE12 5RD, United Kingdom; [c] Academic Division of Child Health, Obstetrics & Gynaecology, School of Medicine, D Floor East Block, Queen's Medical Centre, The University of Nottingham, Derby Road, Nottingham, NG7 2UH, United Kingdom
* Corresponding author. Robinson Institute, University of Adelaide, Ground Floor, Norwich Centre, 55 King William Street, North Adelaide, SA 5006, Australia.
E-mail address: viv.perry@adelaide.edu.au

respectively.[1,2] With 90% of these offspring born alive, this is considered a preventable welfare issue[1] and a high economic burden to the livestock industry.

It is well established that in utero environment[3] affects ruminant progeny health and welfare. This phenomenon is known as fetal programming and is contingent upon the particularly long gestation period in ruminants during which physiologic systems develop, such that at birth, the ontogeny of these systems is complete. The effects of this fetal programming in the neonate may be mediated by epigenetic modifications that regulate gene expression in both the placenta and the fetus[4] (**Fig. 1**). These epigenetic modifications may occur as early as embryogenesis[5] through to late gestation.[6] The placenta mediates fetal supply of nutrients, hormones, and oxygen[7,8] with both the placenta and the fetus responding to maternal perturbations in a sexually dimorphic manner.[9,10] This dimorphism has significant consequences because survival in the male fetus, during gestation and at birth, is reduced[11] compared with the female fetus.

Significantly for this review, many of the contributing factors associated with increased risk of neonatal mortality, that is, premature birth,[12] birth weight,[13] dystocia,[14,15] and poor adaptation to the postnatal environment,[16,17] are consequent to the prevailing prenatal environment.[3] Moreover, neonatal appetite, adiposity, and

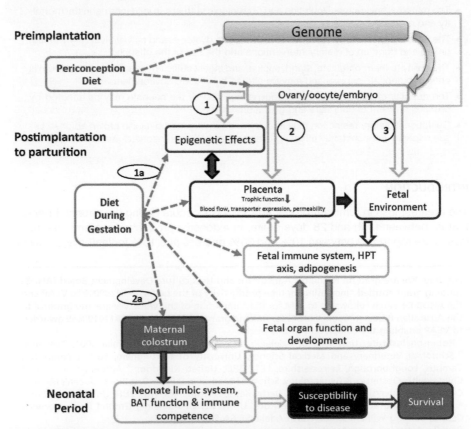

Fig. 1. (*1*) Fetoplacental unit responds to nutrient intake. (*1a*) Epigenetic changes in fetoplacental genes in response to nutrition. (*2*) Blood flow to the placenta and transporter changes affect placental permeability and function. (*2a*) Gestational diet alters colostrum quality (Immunoglobulins) and quantity. (*3*) Placental hormonal output modulates fetal environment.

immune function may be influenced by gestational diet in cattle[18,19] and sheep.[20] In this review, the authors address those aspects of neonatal mortality affected by fetal programming with particular reference to the bovine.

BIRTH WEIGHT, DYSTOCIA, AND NEONATAL SURVIVAL

Dystocia is the main cause of neonatal calf mortality,[14,21] either directly or indirectly via decreased vigor.[22] Calves that survive dystocia are reported to experience lower passive immunity transfer and increased risk of postnatal morbidity and mortality[23] and display higher indicators of physiologic stress.[11]

The incidence of dystocia in nulliparous beef heifers is higher than in multiparous cows,[13,24] despite birth weight of first parity progeny generally being lower.[25] High birth weight sufficient to cause dystocia is the major cause of neonatal calf loss.[22,26] A disproportionately large calf is the major contributor to dystocia in heifers,[23,24] with calf birth weight[27] and heifer size[15] considered the primary factors causing this fetal-maternal disproportion. In growing heifers, particularly those calving at 2 years of age, there is greater nutrient competition between the dam and rapidly developing fetus. They are effectively an adolescent[28] and display a greater response to dietary restriction compared with adults[29] similar to that observed in the ewe.[30] However, both low- and high-birth-weight extremes may be caused by dietary perturbations during gestation with extremely low-birth-weight calves also showing increased susceptibility to morbidity in cold climates[31] as observed in the lamb. Intriguingly, cold climate temperatures during gestation may be sufficient in themselves to reduce birth weight.[32]

As illustrated in **Table 1**, the timing of dietary interventions impacts the observed effect on birth weight: Interventions imposed before 100 days postconception (dpc), although causing greater effects on fetal organ development,[33] generally result in similar birth weights at term.[34] Nutrient restriction during the second trimester, however, may have the greatest influence on calf birth weight[2,29,35] sufficient to influence dystocia and thereby survival in the neonate.

Dietary interventions aimed at reducing birth weight and dystocia during the third trimester have produced varied responses.[25,36–39] This variation appears to be dependent on the severity of maternal weight loss.[29] However, this effect is generally not associated with reductions in dystocia perhaps due to increased length of second-stage labor.[15] In contrast, studies in sheep show maternal undernutrition[40] or overnutrition[41] in late pregnancy may reduce lamb birth weight with this effect commensurate with the level of weight change in the ewe.[3]

There is a sex-specific variation in dystocia rates in cattle, with greater occurrence typically associated with male offspring experiencing increased dystocia, neonatal morbidity, and mortality concomitant with their heavier birth weight[48] and placental dysfunction.[11] This effect is commensurate with the observed greater effect of early gestational perturbation to male fetal and placental growth and uterine hemodynamics.[9,10,28] Reductions in birth weight have also been observed following heat stress[49] and individual dietary nutrient restrictions.[2,45,50,51] Protein supplementation in mid to late gestation has been reported to have either no effect on birth weight[39,45,52,53] or an increased calf birth weight when cows graze low-quality winter pasture.[51] Protein supplementation during the second trimester in *Bos indicus* heifers increased birth weight by 8% while increasing dystocia rates 3-fold.[2]

Table 1 illustrates that the effects of maternal nutrient restriction during gestation on calf birth weight and dystocia vary dependent on age and parity of the dams studied, the nutritional regimens, and the timing of perturbation.[2,14,38] This table effectively clarifies the importance of timing and duration of gestational intervention,

Table 1
The effects of gestational dietary interventions on fetal development, birth weight, and dystocia

Refs	Dam Parity (Hf = Heifer & C = Cow)	n =	Period of Intervention (Days to Conception) Treatment	Effects of Treatment on (L Compare with H or Control)					Pregnancy Stage/Trimester (Days) Relative to Conception			
				Sex	Placenta	Fetal	Birth Weight	Dystocia	Pre (−60 d)	First (0–90 d)	Second (90–180 d)	Third (>181 d)
Hernandez-Medrano et al,[9] 2015; Copping et al,[28] 2014	Hf	120	−60 d to 23 d & 24–90 d 2 × 2 Factorial design	L = 7% CP[b] vs H = 14% CP[b]	Y (M > F)	↑ MUA blood flow	↓ wt (98 d) & ↓ CRL (32 d)	=	=			
Mossa et al,[33] 2013	Hf	23	−11 d to 110 d RA: 110 d to term	Female only[a] L = 60% E Mreq[a] vs H = 120% E Mreq[a] RA: 140% E Mreq[a]		NA	NA	=	=			
Sullivan et al,[8] 2009; Micke et al,[2] 2010	Hf	120	0–93 d & 94–180 d 2 × 2 Factorial design	L = 4% CP[b] vs H = 13% CP[b]	Y	NA	↓ CRL (36 d)	= (1st) ↓ (2nd)				
Miguel-Pacheco et al,[35] 2016	Hf	80	14–90 d & 90–180 d 2 × 2 Factorial design	L = 6% CP[b] & vs H = 16% CP[b] (RA)	Y (F > M)	NA	NA	↓				
Meyer et al,[42] 2010; Vonnahme et al,[43] 2007	C	40	30–125 d with RA: 125–220 d	Female only[a] L = 68% Mreq (9.9% CP) vs Ct = 100% Mreq (12% CP) RA: 13.2% CP	NA	↓ wt (cotyl + carunc) ↓ vascularity (cotyl)	↓ wt (125 d) but = (after RA) & ↑ GI tract	NA	NA			

Study		n	Intervention period	Diet				
Perry et al,[44] 1999	Hf	16	42–90 d & 90–180 d	L = 7% CP[b] vs H = 14% CP[b] 2 × 2 Factorial design	NA	↑ cotyl wt (LL/LH) & ↑ troph vol (LH/HL)	NA	=
Anthony et al,[39] 1986	Hf	59	75 d to term	L = 81% Mreq vs H = 141% Mreq (CPreq)	NA	NA	NA	=
Freetly et al,[29] 2000	C	144	90 d to term	28 kg wt loss	NA	NA	↓	NA
Summers et al,[45] 2015	Hf	114	167–226 d	Isocaloric and isonitrogenous with L = 34% RUP vs H = 59% RUP RA	N	NA	=	NA
Bellows et al,[46] 1978	Hf & C		190 d to term	L = 3.2–3.4 kg TDN vs H = 6.3–6.4 kg TDN	NA	NA	↓ (Hf only)	NA
Tudor,[47] 1972	Hf & C	79 (Hf = 36 & C = 43)	180 d to term	L = 12.5% CP[a] vs H = 14.4% CP[a]	NA	NA	↓ pregnancy length	NA
Corah et al,[48] 1975	Hf	59	180 d to term	L = 65% Mreq[a] vs H = 100% Mreq[a]	N/A	↓ (2 kg)	N/A	=

Abbreviations: ↑, increase; ↓, decrease; =, no effect; carunc, caruncle; cotyl, cotyledon; CP, crude protein; CRL, crown-rump length; E, energy; F, female; Green block, intervention period; H, high; L, low; M, male; Mreq, maintenance requirement according to NRC(^{a}) or ARC(^{b}); MUA, mid-uterine artery; NA, variable not measured/tested; N, no; RA, realimentation; RUP, rumen undegradable protein; troph, trophectoderm; white block, realimentation period; wt, weight; 1st, first trimester of pregnancy; 2nd, second trimester of pregnancy; Y, yes.

severity of the intervention, and sex of the offspring in the neonatal phenotype at birth.

NEONATAL ADAPTATION

Neonatal survival is dependent on the ability of the neonate to adapt rapidly to the ex utero environment. Sequentially, the ability to thermoregulate, stand, suckle, and ingest sufficient quantities of colostrum in the first hours of life is required.[54]

A calf's ability to thermoregulate is largely determined by the function of brown adipose tissue (BAT). BAT constitutes only 2% of body fat at birth but provides 50% of thermogenic response as nonshivering thermogenesis.[55] Adipogenesis, as with myogenesis and organogenesis, is complete in cattle and sheep before birth as it is in the human.[56] It is not surprising therefore that adipose tissue, including BAT, is significantly influenced by prenatal diet.[18,57,58] Adipose tissue has an important regulatory and homeostatic function particularly in the neonate.[59] BAT produces heat at 300 W/kg compared with 1 W/kg of in all other tissues,[60] by expressing a BAT-specific gene called uncoupling protein 1 (UCP1), which dramatically increases fuel oxidation.[61] One critical process in ensuring maximal activation of BAT is intracellular conversion of the thyroid hormone thyroxine to its active form, triiodothyronine (T3), by the enzyme 5′monodeiodinase type 2.[62] Thermoregulation and overall neonatal survival are influenced by the interaction between thyroid hormones, deiodinases, and BAT.[63] Restricted maternal diet during pregnancy has been shown to increase levels of thyroid hormones in the neonate, which may be able to upregulate UCP1 expression, acting to increase thermogenesis.[10] This increased thermogenesis may be a mean by which low-birth-weight calves can increase heat production. Interestingly, in rats, low-birth-weight offspring have raised UCP1 compared with normal-sized litter mates.[64]

As the fetal thyroid gland differentiates between 75 and 90 dpc, maternal dietary restriction during early gestation may reset the physiology of the hypothalamic–pituitary–thyroid (HPT) axis by altering ontogeny of the thyroid.[65] This altered ontogeny may act to increase free T3 (FT3) levels observed in the neonatal calf[10] and lamb.[66] As reported in lambs,[66,67] this increased FT3 may contribute to the "catch-up growth" of these low-birth-weight calves,[68] particularly because FT3 was positively correlated with average daily weight gain and fetal growth rate in calves in this study.[10]

Feeding behavior at birth is fundamental to calf survival, with the licking of the cow first stimulating the calf to stand and suckle.[69] This licking initiates the bond between mother and offspring.[70] Dairy calves take an average of 90 minutes to stand after birth and up to 6 hours to suckle for the first time,[69,71,72] whereas beef calves take up to 2 hours.[73] This time to first standing influences colostrum intake within the first 24 hours after birth.[74,75] Calves that take longer to stand will take longer to suckle,[71] potentially delaying the passive transfer of immunity and the provision of energy in the initial hours after birth.

Cows with highly responsive calves are more likely to provide maternal care,[76] which is important in free-ranging animals. The ability of a calf to stand and suckle is influenced by calf birth weight, sex, and ease of calving.[11] Periconception and first-trimester restricted protein intake in heifers has been shown to affect neonatal behavior of offspring.[77] Calves from heifers fed a low protein diet before conception showed higher duration of suckling behavior[77] sufficient to increase milk output.[78,79] Low-birth-weight calves have been reported to stimulate nursing bouts more frequently than calves with a higher birth weight.[76] This enhanced appetite may be prenatally programmed as neural pathways that are pivotal to appetite and voluntary food intake, which develop early in fetal ruminant life.[80] Gestational dietary restriction alters gene expression for primary appetite regulating hypothalamic neuropeptides[81] and thereby appetite in the neonate.

NEONATAL IMMUNE FUNCTION

Ontogeny of the bovine immune response is parallel to the human because of similar gestational periods[82] with differentiation complete by the end of the first trimester. Three critical windows of vulnerability exist during the first trimester of gestation[83]: the period of embryonic stem cell formation, fetal liver development as the primary hematopoietic organ, and colonization and establishment of bone marrow and thymus. In the calf, lymphoid development of the thymus is complete at 42 dpc, with the spleen structurally present at 55 dpc, and peripheral and mesenteric lymph nodes at 60 dpc and 100 dpc, respectively. Thymic and splenic indices reach maximal values from 205 dpc. Therefore, the thymus has been suggested as the mediator of the effects of early gestational perturbation upon immune function in neonates.[84,85] Copping and colleagues[84] report that fetal thymus size and antibiotic use in the neonate may be altered by protein restriction early in gestation concomitant with effects upon colostral immunoglobulins.[10]

Allied with BAT's role in thermogenesis is the relationship with the function of neonatal immune and lymph systems. Prenatal dietary restriction may alter both thyroid function (as above) and diminish BAT capacity,[86] concomitantly effecting lymphoid atrophy.[87] Lymphoid tissues are susceptible to in utero perturbations early in gestation as thymic differentiation occurs by 42 dpc in the calf (similar to the human[88]) with other lymphoid structures present by 100 dpc.[82] BAT depots surround lymphoid tissues (including the thymus) in neonatal calves and lambs. It is proposed that they act not only as a dedicated lipid resource fueling immune activation in lymph nodes[89] but also to provide key fatty-acid, cellular, and adipokine immunoregulatory material that supports and regulates local immunity.[90] BAT located around the prescapular lymph node and sternal areas leading to the thymus is abundant in the neonatal calf[91] as it is in the lamb.[58] This BAT depot exhibits a different gene expression profile to perirenal BAT but may equally be susceptible to in utero intervention.[58,92] Interestingly, cattle breeds with better neonatal cold survival have increased expression of genes associated with BAT and immune function.[93,94]

Late gestational stressors, such as heat,[95] disease, drought,[21] or even dystocia,[11] may also affect immune function in the neonatal calf. The mechanisms driving this effect may include a reduction in food intake during the prenatal stress period. Nutritional supplementation with methionine, in combination with a high-energy diet, during the last trimester of pregnancy causes a decreased inflammatory response in the neonatal calf, by modulation of cellular responses.[96] These stress or nutritional interventions are thought to affect the calf via changes in cellular interactions with pathogens (CD18 and CD14) and changes in acute phase cytokines and pathogen recognition.[54]

Acquisition of passive immunity via colostral immunoglobulins in the first 24 hours of life[97–99] is required for calf survival.[100–102] The quantity of colostral immunoglobulin ingested is affected by dam age, prenatal ambient temperature,[96] and gestational diet.[103–105] Timing, severity, and period of prenatal intervention modify the observed affect.

Cows restricted from 90 dpc to term show immunoglobulin G (IgG) concentrations double that compared with cattle on a high plane of nutrition.[106] The latter effect may occur as the cow attempts to maintain transfer of passive immunity in the face of restricted diet.[106] Increased ambient temperatures late in gestation may decrease colostral IgG and IgA.[105]

Primiparous heifers may produce less colostrum with lower concentration of immunoglobulins compared with multiparous cows.[104] Calves from such heifers, however, have been reported to have higher antibody concentrations despite lower levels of immunoglobulins being present in the colostrum.[107] This adaptation may be associated with necessity considering the lower birth weight of primiparous heifer calves.

SUMMARY

The authors have illustrated that the prenatal period influences neonatal mortality. Nutrient restriction, protein restriction, elevated ambient temperature, or a stress event during gestation may affect neonatal survival. This effect upon the neonate occurs by influencing a) Dystocia, both via increasing birth weight and placental dysfunction; (b) Thermoregulation, both via altering the amount of BAT and its ability to function via effects on the HPT axis; (c) Modification of the developing immune system and its symbiotic nutrient sources; (d) Modification of maternal and neonatal behavior. A lack of attention to these critical windows during prenatal life is hazardous to the commercial production of live calves.

REFERENCES

1. Mee J. Why do so many calves die on modern dairy farms and what can we do about calf welfare in the future? Animals 2013;3(4):1036.
2. Micke GC, Sullivan TM, Soares Magalhaes RJ, et al. Heifer nutrition during early- and mid-pregnancy alters fetal growth trajectory and birth weight. Anim Reprod Sci 2010;117(1–2):1–10.
3. Sinclair KD, Rutherford KMD, Wallace JM, et al. Epigenetics and developmental programming of welfare and production traits in farm animals. Reprod Fertil Dev 2016;28(10):1443–78.
4. Vickaryous N, Whitelaw E. The role of early embryonic environment on epigenotype and phenotype. Reprod Fertil Dev 2005;17(3):335–40.
5. Bermejo-Alvarez P, Rizos D, Lonergan P, et al. Transcriptional sexual dimorphism in elongating bovine embryos: implications for XCI and sex determination genes. Reproduction 2011;141(6):801–8.
6. Skibiel AL, Peñagaricano F, Amorín R, et al. In utero heat stress alters the offspring epigenome. Sci Rep 2018;8(1):14609.
7. Vaughan OR, Sferruzzi-Perri AN, Coan PM, et al. Environmental regulation of placental phenotype: implications for fetal growth. Reprod Fertil Dev 2011; 24(1):80–96.
8. Sullivan TM, Micke GC, Magalhaes RS, et al. Dietary protein during gestation affects circulating indicators of placental function and fetal development in heifers. Placenta 2009;30(4):348–54.
9. Hernandez-Medrano JH, Copping KJ, Hoare A, et al. Gestational dietary protein is associated with sex specific decrease in blood flow, fetal heart growth and post-natal blood pressure of progeny. PLoS One 2015;10(4):e0125694.
10. Micke GC, Sullivan TM, Kennaway DJ, et al. Maternal endocrine adaptation throughout pregnancy to nutrient manipulation: consequences for sexually dimorphic programming of thyroid hormones and development of their progeny. Theriogenology 2015;83(4):604–15.
11. Barrier AC, Haskell MJ, Birch S, et al. The impact of dystocia on dairy calf health, welfare, performance and survival. Vet J 2013;195(1):86–90.
12. Bloomfield FH, Oliver MH, Hawkins P, et al. A periconceptional nutritional origin for noninfectious preterm birth. Science 2003;300(5619):606.
13. Morris CA, Bennett GL, Baker RL, et al. Birth weight, dystocia and calf mortality in some New Zealand beef breeding herds. J Anim Sci 1986;62:327–43.

14. Hickson RE, Morris ST, Kenyon PR, et al. Dystocia in beef heifers: a review of genetic and nutritional influences. N Z Vet J 2006;54(6):256–64.
15. Zaborski D, Grzesiak W, Szatkowska I, et al. Factors affecting dystocia in cattle. Reprod Domest Anim 2009;44(3):540–51.
16. Kleemann DO, Kelly JM, Rudiger SR, et al. Effect of periconceptional nutrition on the growth, behaviour and survival of the neonatal lamb. Anim Reprod Sci 2015; 160:12–22.
17. Carstens GE, Johnson DE, Holland MD, et al. Effects of prepartum protein nutrition and birth weight on basal metabolism in bovine neonates. J Anim Sci 1987; 65:745–51.
18. Micke GC, Sullivan TM, McMillen IC, et al. Heifer nutrient intake during early- and mid-gestation programs adult offspring adiposity and mRNA expression of growth-related genes in adipose depots. Reproduction 2011;141(5):697–706.
19. Sullivan TM, Micke GC, Perry VEA. Influences of diet during gestation on potential postpartum reproductive performance and milk production of beef heifers. Theriogenology 2009;72(9):1202–14.
20. McMillen IC, MacLaughlin SM, Muhlhausler BS, et al. Developmental origins of adult health and disease: the role of periconceptional and foetal nutrition. Basic Clin Pharmacol Toxicol 2008;102(2):82–9.
21. Arnott G, Roberts D, Rooke JA, et al. Board invited review: the importance of the gestation period for welfare of calves: maternal stressors and difficult births. J Anim Sci 2012;90(13):5021–34.
22. Mee JF. Prevalence and risk factors for dystocia in dairy cattle: a review. Vet J 2008;176:93–101.
23. Rice LE. Dystocia-related risk factors. Vet Clin North Am Food Anim Pract 1994; 10:53–68.
24. Philipsson J. Calving performance and calf mortality. Livest Prod Sci 1976;3: 319–31.
25. Bellows RA, Short RE. Effects of precalving feed level on birthweight, calving difficulty and subsequent fertility. J Anim Sci 1978;46:1522–8.
26. Comerford JW, Bertrand JK, Benyshek LL, et al. Reproductive rates, birth weight, calving ease and 24-h calf survival in a four-breed diallel among Simmental, Limousin, Polled Hereford and Brahman beef cattle. J Anim Sci 1987;64:65–76.
27. Arthur PF, Archer JA, Melville GJ. Factors influencing dystocia and prediction of dystocia in Angus heifers selected for yearling growth rate. Aust J Agric Res 2000;51:147–53.
28. Copping KJ, Hoare A, Callaghan M, et al. Fetal programming in 2-year-old calving heifers: peri-conception and first trimester protein restriction alters fetal growth in a gender-specific manner. Anim Prod Sci 2014;54(9):1333–7.
29. Freetly HC, Ferrell CL, Jenkins TG. Timing of realimentation of mature cows that were feed-restricted during pregnancy influences calf birth weights and growth rates. J Anim Sci 2000;78:2790–6.
30. Wallace J, Bourke D, Da Silva P, et al. Nutrient partitioning during adolescent pregnancy. Reproduction 2001;122(3):347–57.
31. Dwyer CM, Bünger L. Factors affecting dystocia and offspring vigour in different sheep genotypes. Prev Vet Med 2012;103(4):257–64.
32. Andreoli K, Minton J, Spire M, et al. Influence of prepartum exposure of beef heifers to winter weather on concentrations of plasma energy-yielding substrates, serum hormones and birth weight of calves. Theriogenology 1988;29: 631–42.

33. Mossa F, Carter F, Walsh SW, et al. Maternal undernutrition in cows impairs ovarian and cardiovascular systems in their offspring. Biol Reprod 2013;88(4): 92, 1-9.

34. Long NM, Prado-Cooper MJ, Krehbiel CR, et al. Effects of nutrient restriction of bovine dams during early gestation on postnatal growth and regulation of plasma glucose. J Anim Sci 2010;88(10):3262–8.

35. Miguel-Pacheco GG, Curtain LD, Rutland C, et al. Increased dietary protein in the second trimester of gestation increases live weight gain and carcass composition in weaner calves to 6 months of age. Animal 2017;11(6):991–9.

36. Rasby RJ, Wettemann RP, Geisert RD, et al. Nutrition, body condition and repro-duction in beef cows: fetal and placental development, and estrogens and pro-gesterone in plasma. J Anim Sci 1990;68:4267–76.

37. Tudor GD. The effect of pre- and post-natal nutrition on the growth of beef cattle. I. The effect of nutrition and parity on the dam on calf birth weight. Aust J Agric Res 1972;23:389–95.

38. Holland MD, Odde KG. Factors affecting calf birth weight: a review. Therioge-nology 1992;38(5):769–98.

39. Anthony RV, Bellows RA, Short RE, et al. Fetal growth of beef calves. I. Effect of prepartum dietary crude protein on birth weight, blood metabolites and steroid hormone concentrations. J Anim Sci 1986;62(5):1363–74.

40. Rooke JA, Arnott G, Dwyer CM, et al. The importance of the gestation period for welfare of lambs: maternal stressors and lamb vigour and wellbeing. J Agric Sci 2014;153(3):497–519.

41. Wallace JM, Milne JS, Aitken RP. The effect of overnourishing singleton-bearing adult ewes on nutrient partitioning to the gravid uterus. Br J Nutr 2005;94(4): 533–9.

42. Meyer AM, Reed JJ, Vonnahme KA, et al. Effects of stage of gestation and nutrient restriction during early to mid-gestation on maternal and fetal visceral organ mass and indices of jejunal growth and vascularity in beef cows1. J Anim Sci 2010;88(7):2410–24.

43. Vonnahme KA, Zhu MJ, Borowicz PP, et al. Effect of early gestational undernu-trition on angiogenic factor expression and vascularity in the bovine placen-tome. J Anim Sci 2007;85(10):2464–72.

44. Perry VE, Norman ST, Owen JA, et al. Low dietary protein during early preg-nancy alters bovine placental development. Anim Reprod Sci 1999;55(1):13–21.

45. Summers AF, Meyer TL, Funston RN. Impact of supplemental protein source offered to primiparous heifers during gestation on I. Average daily gain, feed intake, calf birth body weight, and rebreeding in pregnant beef heifers. J Anim Sci 2015;93(4):1865–70.

46. Bellows RA, Carr JB, Patterson DJ, et al. Effects of ration protein content on dystocia and reproduction in beef heifers. Journal of Animal Science 1978; 47(Supl 1):175–7.

47. Tudor G. Effect of pre- and post- natal nutrition on the growth of beef cattle I. The effect of nutrition and parity of the dam on calf birth weight. Aust J Agric Res 1972;23(3):389–95.

48. Corah LR, Dunn TG, Kaltenbach CC. Influence of prepartum nutrition on the reproductive performance of beef females and the performance of their prog-eny. J Anim Sci 1975;41(3):819–24.

49. Monteiro APA, Tao S, Thompson IMT, et al. In utero heat stress decreases calf survival and performance through the first lactation. J Dairy Sci 2016;99(10): 8443–50.

50. Radunz AE, Fluharty FL, Day ML, et al. Prepartum dietary energy source fed to beef cows: I. Effects on pre- and postpartum cow performance. J Anim Sci 2010;88(8):2717–28.

51. Larson DM, Martin JL, Adams DC, et al. Winter grazing system and supplementation during late gestation influence performance of beef cows and steer progeny. J Anim Sci 2009;87(3):1147–55.

52. Martin JL, Vonnahme KA, Adams DC, et al. Effects of dam nutrition on growth and reproductive performance of heifer calves. J Anim Sci 2007;85(3):841–7.

53. Stalker LA, Adams DC, Klopfenstein TJ, et al. Effects of pre- and postpartum nutrition on reproduction in spring calving cows and calf feedlot performance. J Anim Sci 2006;84(9):2582–9.

54. Tao S, Monteiro AP, Thompson IM, et al. Effect of late-gestation maternal heat stress on growth and immune function of dairy calves. J Dairy Sci 2012; 95(12):7128–36.

55. Alexander G, Williams D. Shivering and nonshivering thermogenesis during summit metabolism in young lambs. J Physiol 1968;198:251–76.

56. Vernon RG. The growth and metabolism of adipocytes. In: Buttery PJ, Haynes NB, Lindsay DB, editors. Control and manipulation of animal growth. London: Butterworths; 1986. p. 67–83.

57. Clarke L, Bryant MJ, Lomax MA, et al. Maternal manipulation of brown adipose tissue and liver development in the ovine fetus during late gestation. Br J Nutr 1997;77:871–83.

58. Fainberg HP, Birtwistle M, Alagal R, et al. Transcriptional analysis of adipose tissue during development reveals depot-specific responsiveness to maternal dietary supplementation. Sci Rep 2018;8:9628.

59. Hausman GJ, Richardson RL. Adipose tissue angiogenesis. J Anim Sci 2004; 82(3):925–34.

60. Power G. Biology of temperature: the mammalian fetus. J Dev Physiol 1989;12: 295–304.

61. Clarke L, Heasman L, Firth K, et al. Influence of route of delivery and ambient temperature on thermoregulation in newborn lambs. Am J Physiol Regul Integr Comp Physiol 1997;272(6 Pt 2):R1931–9.

62. Bianco AC, Silva JE. Intracellular conversion of thyroxine to triiodothyronine is required for the optimal thermogenic function of brown adipose tissue. J Clin Invest 1987;79:295–300.

63. Symonds ME, Clarke L. Influence of thyroid hormones and temperature on adipose tissue development and lung maturation. Proc Nutr Soc 1996;55:567–75.

64. Dumortier O, Roger E, Pisani DF, et al. Age-dependent control of energy homeostasis by brown adipose tissue in progeny subjected to maternal diet-induced fetal programming. Diabetes 2017;66(3):627–39.

65. Johnsen L, Lyckegaard NB, Khanal P, et al. Fetal over- and undernutrition differentially program thyroid axis adaptability in adult sheep. Endocr Connect 2018; 7(5):777–90.

66. De Blasio MJ, Gatford KL, Robinson JS, et al. Placental restriction alters circulating thyroid hormone in the young lamb postnatally. Am J Physiol 2006;291: R1016–24.

67. Hernandez MV, Etta KM, Reineke EP, et al. Thyroid function in the prenatal and neonatal bovine. J Anim Sci 1972;34(5):780–5.

68. Micke GC, Sullivan TM, Gatford KL, et al. Nutrient intake in the bovine during early and mid-gestation causes sex-specific changes in progeny plasma

IGF-I, liveweight, height and carcass traits. Anim Reprod Sci 2010;121(3–4): 208–17.

69. Jensen MB. Behaviour around the time of calving in dairy cows. Appl Anim Behav Sci 2012;139(3–4):195–202.

70. Johnsen JF, de Passille AM, Mejdell CM, et al. The effect of nursing on the cow–calf bond. Appl Anim Behav Sci 2015;163:50–7.

71. Ventorp M, Michanek P. Cow-calf behaviour in relation to first suckling. Res Vet Sci 1991;51(1):6–10.

72. von Keyserlingk MAG, Weary DM. Maternal behavior in cattle. Horm Behav 2007;52(1):106–13.

73. Lidfors LM, Moran D, Jung J, et al. Behaviour at calving and choice of calving place in cattle kept in different environments. Applied Animal Behaviour Science 1994;42(1):11–28.

74. Godden S. Colostrum management for dairy calves. Vet Clin North Am Food Anim Pract 2008;24(1):19–39.

75. Homerosky ER, Timsit E, Pajor EA, et al. Predictors and impacts of colostrum consumption by 4h after birth in newborn beef calves. Vet J 2017;228:1–6.

76. Stehulova I, Spinka M, Sarova R, et al. Maternal behaviour in beef cows is individually consistent and sensitive to cow body condition, calf sex and weight. Appl Anim Behav Sci 2013;144(3–4):89–97.

77. Miguel-Pacheco G, Hernandez-Medrano J, Keisler DH, et al. Is maternal behaviour affected by peri-conception diet? Paper presented at: Proceedings of the 50th Congress of the International Society for Applied Ethology 2016. Edinburgh, United Kingdom.

78. Bar-Peled U, Maltz E, Bruckental I, et al. Relationship between frequent milking or suckling in early lactation and milk production of high producing dairy cows. J Dairy Sci 1995;78(12):2726–36.

79. Wall EH, McFadden TB. The milk yield response to frequent milking in early lactation of dairy cows is locally regulated. J Dairy Sci 2007;90(2):716–20.

80. Muhlhausler BS, Adam CL, Findlay PA, et al. Increased maternal nutrition alters development of the appetite-regulating network in the brain. FASEB J 2006;20: 1257–9.

81. Begum G, Stevens A, Smith EB, et al. Epigenetic changes in fetal hypothalamic energy regulating pathways are associated with maternal undernutrition and twinning. FASEB J 2012;26(4):1694–703.

82. Schultz RD, Dunne HW, Heist CE. Ontogeny of the bovine immune response. Infect Immun 1973;7(6):981–91.

83. Merlot E, Couret D, Otten W. Prenatal stress, fetal imprinting and immunity. Brain Behav Immun 2008;22(1):42–51.

84. Copping KJ, DL, Flynn R, et al. Sex specific effects of early gestational diet upon the developing immune system. Proceedings 2015 Annual Scientific Meeting of the Endocrine Society of Australia and the Society for Reproductive Biology. 23 – 26th August 2015. Adelaide, Australia. Society for Reproductive Biology; 31.

85. Cronjé PB. Foetal programming of immune competence. Aust J Exp Agr 2003; 43(12):1427–30.

86. Jones CT, Lafeber HN, Rolph TP, et al. Studies on the growth of the fetal guinea pig. The effects of nutritional manipulation on prenatal growth and plasma somatomedin activity and insulin-like growth factor concentrations. J Dev Physiol 1990;13(4):189–97.

87. Cromi A, Ghezzi F, Raffaelli R, et al. Ultrasonographic measurement of thymus size in IUGR fetuses: a marker of the fetal immunoendocrine response to malnutrition. Ultrasound Obstet Gynecol 2009;33(4):421–6.

88. Chandra RK. Nutrition and the immune system: an introduction. Am J Clin Nutr 1997;66(2):460S–3S.

89. Pond WG, Maurer RR, Mersmann H, et al. Response of fetal and newborn piglets to maternal protein restriction during early or late pregnancy. Growth Dev Aging 1992;56(3):115–27.

90. Pond CM. Adipose tissue and the immune system. Prostaglandins Leukot Essent Fatty Acids 2005;73(1):17–30.

91. Pickwell ND. Molecular profiles of brown, 'brite' and white bovine neonate adipose tissues [Masters]. Nottingham: School of Veterinary Medicine and Science, University of Nottingham; 2013.

92. Henry BA, Pope M, Birtwistle M, et al. Ontogeny and thermogenic role for sternal fat in female sheep. Endocrinology 2017;158(7):2212–25.

93. Cundiff LV, MacNeil MD, Gregory KE, et al. Between- and within-breed genetic analysis of calving traits and survival to weaning in beef cattle. J Anim Sci 1986; 63(1):27–33.

94. Smith SB, Carstens GE, Randel RD, et al. Brown adipose tissue development and metabolism in ruminants. J Anim Sci 2004;82(3):942–54.

95. Strong RA, Silva EB, Cheng HW, et al. Acute brief heat stress in late gestation alters neonatal calf innate immune functions1. J Dairy Sci 2015;98(11):7771–83.

96. Jacometo CB, Alharthi AS, Zhou Z, et al. Maternal supply of methionine during late pregnancy is associated with changes in immune function and abundance of microRNA and mRNA in Holstein calf polymorphonuclear leukocytes. J Dairy Sci 2018;101(9):8146–58.

97. Ball PJ, Peters AR. Reproduction in cattle. 3rd edition. United kingdom: Wiley Online Library; 2004.

98. Porter P. Immunoglobulins in bovine mammary secretions: quantitative changes in early lactation and absorption by the neonatal calf. Immunology 1972;23(2): 225.

99. Jaster EH. Evaluation of quality, quantity, and timing of colostrum feeding on immunoglobulin G1 absorption in jersey calves. J Dairy Sci 2005;88(1):296–302.

100. Robison JD, Stott GH, DeNise SK. Effects of passive immunity on growth and survival in the dairy heifer1,2. J Dairy Sci 1988;71(5):1283–7.

101. McEwan AD, Fisher EW, Selman IE. Observations on the immune globulin levels of neonatal calves and their relationship to disease. J Comp Pathol 1970;80(2): 259–65.

102. Dewell RD, Hungerford LL, Keen JE, et al. Association of neonatal serum immunoglobulin G1 concentration with health and performance in beef calves. J Am Vet Med Assoc 2006;228(6):914–21.

103. Hough R, McCarthy F, Kent H, et al. Influence of nutritional restriction during late gestation on production measures and passive immunity in beef cattle. J Anim Sci 1990;68(9):2622–7.

104. McGee M, Drennan MJ, Caffrey PJ. Effect of age and nutrient restriction pre partum on beef suckler cow serum immunoglobulin concentrations, colostrum yield, composition and immunoglobulin concentration and immune status of their progeny. Irish Journal of Agricultural and Food Research 2006;45(2): 157–71.

105. Nardone A, Lacetera N, Bernabucci U, et al. Composition of colostrum from dairy heifers exposed to high air temperatures during late pregnancy and the early postpartum period. J Dairy Sci 1997;80(5):838–44.
106. Shell T, Early R, Carpenter J, et al. Prepartum nutrition and solar radiation in beef cattle: II. Residual effects on postpartum milk yield, immunoglobulin, and calf growth. J Anim Sci 1995;73(5):1303–9.
107. Shivley CB, Lombard JE, Urie NJ, et al. Preweaned heifer management on US dairy operations: Part II. Factors associated with colostrum quality and passive transfer status of dairy heifer calves. J Dairy Sci 2018;101(10):9185–98.

Developmental Programming and Growth of Livestock Tissues for Meat Production

Paul L. Greenwood, PhD[a],*, Alan W. Bell, PhD[b]

KEYWORDS

- Fetus • Maternal nutrition • Developmental programming • Carcass • Meat quality
- Feed efficiency

KEY POINTS

- Severe fetal growth retardation due to restricted maternal nutrition and/or placental limitations, particularly during late pregnancy, may limit postnatal growth, resulting in livestock that are smaller for age and take longer to reach market weights.
- Differences in efficiency and carcass characteristics of livestock restricted in growth early in life are mostly explained by differences due to size of animals and normal allometric tissue growth patterns; hence differences may no longer be evident at equivalent weights.
- Meat quality seems to be relatively little affected by maternal nutrition and altered fetal growth compared with other postnatal production and processing factors. However, supplementation of grazing pregnant cows with protein during late pregnancy may enhance marbling.
- Management of breeding animals to optimize reproductive rates and efficiency to weaning should ensure minimal adverse effects of developmental programming for growth, efficiency, and meat production from ruminant livestock.

INTRODUCTION

During fetal life, environmental influences on development and growth are mediated through the pregnant dam, before more direct environmental influences on the offspring as postnatal life progresses toward weaning. Influences on development during early life can have long-term consequences for the development and growth trajectories of the body tissues, including bone, muscle, and fat. These early life influences on the development of these tissues may affect the efficiency of meat production and acceptance of meat purchased and eaten by the consumer.

Disclosure: The authors have nothing to disclose.
[a] NSW Department of Primary Industries, Armidale Livestock Industries Centre, University of New England, Armidale, New South Wales 2351, Australia; [b] Department of Animal Science, Cornell University, Ithaca, NY 14853-4801, USA
* Corresponding author.
E-mail address: paul.greenwood@dpi.nsw.gov.au

This article briefly describes the regulation of growth and development of fetal ruminant livestock, with emphasis on nutritional regulation of development of the carcass tissues and consequences for production of meat. The importance of developmental programming in the context of productivity, efficiency, and profitability of beef production systems are briefly discussed. If appropriate, some consequences of fetal and preweaning development are compared. The reader is also referred to earlier reviews on the growth of ruminant livestock fetuses[1] and on the developmental programming of growth, efficiency, and the carcass tissues for ruminant meat production.[2-5]

REGULATION OF FETAL CARCASS TISSUE DEVELOPMENT

The reader is referred to overviews of the biology of carcass tissue development during embryonic and fetal life[4,6] and of metabolism and growth during fetal life.[1,4,7]

Most growth of livestock fetuses occurs during the final third of gestation when fetal growth becomes increasingly susceptible to external influences, particularly nutrient availability and intake by the dam. However, the phase of rapid placental growth precedes that of the fetus, and factors such as nutrition and heat stress can alter growth of the placenta during early pregnancy to midpregnancy, which increasingly constrains fetal growth during the final third of pregnancy as term approaches.[1] Similarly, the size of the placenta constrains growth of fetuses within litters, resulting in lower birthweights with increasing litter size, as evidenced in twin and higher multiples, due to a smaller placenta with fewer placentomes per fetus.[8]

Developmental programming can occur as a result of fetal growth constraint, which becomes quantitatively more significant during later pregnancy, and/or can occur due to altered development not necessarily accompanied by substantially altered fetal growth.[4] The latter is more likely during embryonic and early fetal development when organogenesis of vital organs occurs and development of the carcass tissues commences. These influences may extend to nutritional and other influences on the dam before mating, with carryover effects on the developing embryo and fetus.

Bone

Ossification in fetal sheep commences at about 35 days in jaw bones and by 41 days in the long-bones, thorax, and other bones of the skull.[9] It is generally recognized that embryonic and fetal development of bone precedes development of skeletal muscle, which precedes development of adipose tissue. Bone has a priority for use of available nutrients compared with the soft carcass tissues,[10] hence fetal bone growth is relatively resistant to the growth-limiting effects of restricted nutrient supply. Fetal bone development in livestock has been briefly reviewed.[6]

Severe fetal growth retardation due to factors such as maternal nutrient restriction and placental insufficiency results in smaller bones but a higher proportion of bone relative to muscle and fat within the fetus and newborn.[4,11] More modest reductions in fetal growth in ewes consuming maintenance levels of pasture or with twins reduced the ratio of fetal bone to muscle during late gestation.[12] Overnutrition of pregnant ewes did not affect bone characteristics at birth.[11]

Although bone has a range of essential functions, and the size of bones are primary determinants of mature size and of growth of skeletal muscle and, hence, meat yield and composition, relatively few studies exist on development of bone in the fetus and the consequences for productivity of livestock during postnatal life.[4] Systematic studies to better elucidate bone development in the fetus and the postnatal consequences of compromised fetal bone development for subsequent growth, efficiency, and meat production are required.

Muscle

Myogenesis in livestock species has been reviewed in detail.[13] Myogenesis is essentially complete in all livestock species before birth. Muscle fibers arise from fusion of embryonic and fetal myoblasts into primary myotubes which differentiate into myofibers, or into secondary myofibers that develop around the surface of primary myotubes. Primary myogenesis commences from about day 32 in sheep, before day 37 in cattle, and from about day 35 in pigs. Secondary myogenesis is evident from about day 38 in sheep, day 90 in cattle, and day 55 in pigs. Myogenesis, which may also include a tertiary phase of myofiber development, is believed to be completed by about day 110 in sheep, day 200 in cattle, and day 90 in pigs; that is, at about 70% to 80% of gestation in each species. The reader is also referred to more recent overviews of myogenesis in the context of postnatal growth and development of livestock.[6,14–16]

Myofiber hypertrophy occurs following the conclusion of the hyperplastic phase of muscle development during myogenesis, due to increased accretion of muscle protein in absolute terms and relative to the number of myonuclei in myofibers.[17] This hypertrophic phase of muscle growth is supported by myosatellite cells, which reside between the basal lamina that surrounds the myofiber. Satellite cell mitotic activity allows incorporation of new myonuclei into myofibers as they grow and is sensitive to the growth-determining effects of nutrient supply to the fetus, as a result of either placental or maternal nutritional influences.[17]

During fetal life, the number of myofibers may be reduced in livestock if the supply of nutrients available to the fetus is severely compromised during myogenesis, resulting in reduced formation of myofibers.[18] A reduction in myofiber number requires severe nutritional insult to the fetus during early pregnancy to midpregnancy, which may result from severe, prolonged maternal nutritional restriction during these phases of pregnancy.[19] Impacts on the fetus may be exacerbated if maternal body reserves are depleted as a result of limited nutrient supply before conception and/or high maternal nutrient demand if lactating. In such cases, the supply of nutrients reaching the fetus may be limited as a result of compromised placental development and/or low concentrations of nutrients in maternal circulation. Placental nutrient restriction due to number of fetuses in well-nourished dams did not result in reduced myofiber number.[17,20] Hence, the consequences of reduced number of placentomes per fetus with increasing litter size become increasingly evident during late pregnancy in sheep,[8] when myogenesis is essentially complete but when myofiber hypertrophy normally commences.[17]

A delay in the commencement of hypertrophy of myofibers following completion of myogenesis may limit postnatal muscle growth potential. This was evident in low-birthweight lambs owing to placental restriction on fetal growth during late pregnancy.[20] These fetal lambs had severely restricted myosatellite cell activity associated with very modest rates of protein accretion in muscle, resulting in a delay in the normal increase in the ratio of muscle protein to DNA in fetal livestock.[17] It is likely that severe, prolonged maternal nutritional restriction would result in a similar outcome, potentially coupled with reduced myofiber number if nutrition of the fetus is also compromised earlier during gestation.

Adipose Tissue

Adipose tissue differentiation in fetal ruminants is evident by midgestation.[21–23] Lipid accretion in adipocytes in ovine fetal subcutaneous and perirenal depots is observable by day 70,[24] at which time macroscopically visible adipose tissue can be dissected from the perirenal-abdominal depot.[21] Dissectible subcutaneous fat is present by day 89 of gestation.[21]

Most adipose depots in ruminant fetuses mainly comprise brown fat,[25] although molecular phenotyping of bovine perirenal adipose during late gestation also indicates the presence of white fat cells with minimal lipid.[26] Perirenal adipose increases in volume,[21] which is apparently due to adipocyte hypertrophy[27] during the final 3 to 4 weeks of gestation in fetal sheep. By contrast, the subcutaneous depot comprises white fat that involutes between about day 115 and birth, resulting in negligible visible amounts at term. Sheep have been shown to have 2% to 3%,[21] cattle less than 2%,[28] and pigs about 0.75%[29] body lipid at birth, after which brown adipose tissue in neonatal ruminants transitions to white adipose tissue.[28,30]

Maternal nutrition may influence development of fetal adipose tissue. Undernutrition of ewes in late pregnancy can reduce fetal fatness[31,32] and abundance of mitochondrial uncoupling protein (UCP)-1,[32] with potential implications for heat production in the neonate. Unrestricted feeding of pregnant ewes during late pregnancy following undernutrition in early pregnancy to midpregnancy increased fetal adiposity and mitochondrial UCP-1 abundance.[32]

Overnutrition of ewes during late pregnancy did not affect fatness of fetal lambs but increased expression of genes associated with adipogenesis and lipogenesis in perirenal adipose tissue.[33,34] Overfeeding ewes before and during pregnancy to a level resulting in maternal obesity increased fetal perirenal adipose mass through midgestation and late gestation.[35,36] Similarly, there was more subcutaneous fat and lipogenic gene expression in perirenal adipose evident during late pregnancy in these fetuses.[36] However, transition from excessive feeding of ewes in early pregnancy to predicted requirements for the pregnant ewe normalized fetal fatness.[37]

Newborn lambs of very low birthweight due to placental insufficiency have reduced absolute amounts of body fat but similar bodyweight-specific mass of adipose tissue compared with their normal birthweight counterparts.[38]

DEVELOPMENTAL PROGRAMMING AND MEAT PRODUCTION
Postnatal Growth

Maternal nutritional restriction during pregnancy resulting in fetal growth retardation can reduce postnatal growth and time to reach market weights.[3,4,39] This reduction is more pronounced if maternal undernutrition encompasses late pregnancy when most fetal growth occurs, as opposed to lesser effects on fetal growth during early pregnancy to midpregnancy.

Cows fed pasture of low quality and availability from 80 days of pregnancy to term that resulted in cow weight loss during pregnancy[40] produced offspring that grew more slowly before weaning (independent of carryover maternal nutritional effects on lactation), at similar rates during backgrounding or grow-out, and more slowly in the feedlot (**Figs. 1** and **2, Table 1**).[3] The net effect was a gradual, continual divergence in liveweight from birth to slaughter at 30 months of age compared with offspring of cows grazing pasture of high availability and quality during pregnancy. At slaughter, the difference between the progeny groups due to maternal nutrition during pregnancy was 16.3 kg in liveweight in cattle weighing 678 kg on average. In these cattle, the effect of birthweight on liveweight at slaughter was 4.4 kg of liveweight per kilogram difference in birthweight.[3] In comparison, cows that grazed within these 2 pasture systems throughout lactation produced offspring that exhibited some compensatory growth during backgrounding and similar feedlot growth rates (see

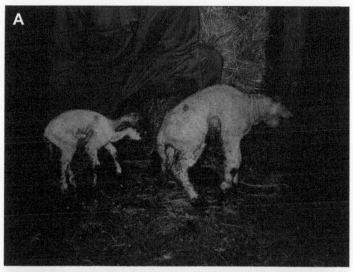

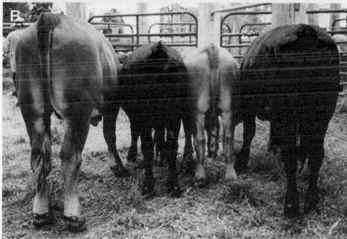

Fig. 1. Consequences of growth variation due to differing factors early in life of ruminants. (*A*) Lambs from the same quadruplet litter varied widely in birthweight (approximately 1.5 kg vs 5 kg) due to differences in the distribution of lambs between uterine horns and the size of their placentas.[8,38] (*B*) Variation in size of calves at the same age postweaning due to factors such as low and high pasture availability during pregnancy and lactation.[3,40]

Figs. 1 and **2, Table 1**).[3] The maternal nutritional effects on offspring during fetal life and during postnatal growth to weaning were additive, and there were no interactions due to genotype of sires for high yield or high marbling (**Fig. 2**).[3]

Similar outcomes to those for cattle have been observed in sheep in relation to postnatal growth following nutritional restriction of ewes during pregnancy and/or offspring intrauterine growth retardation, with lambs exhibiting reduced or similar growth rates to market weights, depending on the severity of restriction during pregnancy.[4]

Postnatal Feed Intake and Efficiency

Feed intake and efficiency seem to be little affected by maternal nutrition during pregnancy and/or fetal growth retardation resulting in reduced birthweight, beyond the

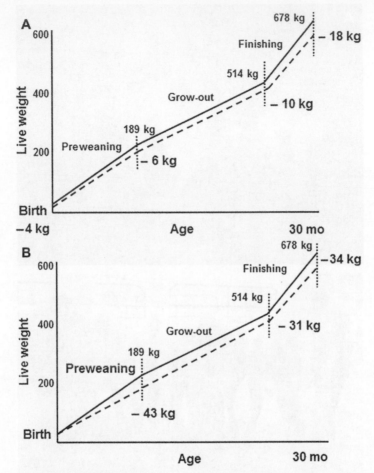

Fig. 2. (*A*) Consequences of poor cow nutrition at pasture during pregnancy resulting in reduced birthweight[3] and (*B*) comparison with consequences of poor cow nutrition at pasture during lactation.[3] Broken and solid lines represent offspring of dams that grazed pasture of low or high nutrient availability and quality, respectively. Negative values are the reductions in liveweight of the poorly nourished compared with the well-nourished offspring.

effects on the size of the offspring.[4] Hence, most of the differences in feedlot intake due to maternal nutrition at pasture during pregnancy and fetal growth of cattle were explained by variation in feedlot entry weights, and differences in feedlot efficiency were not evident (**Table 2**).[4,41] Differences in weaning weight due to maternal nutrition at pasture during lactation affected feedlot intake and feed conversion ratio; however, these were also due only to differences in feedlot entry weight (see **Table 2**).

In sheep, neither birthweight, severely restricted nutrition during early pregnancy to midpregnancy, nor restricted dietary energy provided to ewes in late pregnancy affected offspring intake or efficiency at ages ranging up to 2 years of age.[42–45] Feeding of ewes at 60% of predicted metabolizable energy (ME) requirements from day 45 to 115 of pregnancy resulted in greater postweaning intake by offspring relative to liveweight.[46] This latter finding may have been influenced by carryover effects of pregnant ewe nutritional treatment on lactation performance, which resulted in lambs of nutritionally restricted ewes being lighter at weaning.

Table 1
Effects of birthweight and weaning weight on liveweight, carcass weight, and retail yield

Trait	Mean	Birthweight (Slope/kg Birthweight)	Weaning Weight (Slope/kg Weaning Weight)
Weaning weight (kg)	189	1.53	NA
Grow-out growth rate (g/d)	585	5.44	−0.51
End grow-out weight (kg)	514	3.02	0.72
Feedlot growth rate (kg/d)	1.55	0.014	NS
Feedlot exit weight (kg)	678	4.39	0.78
Hot carcass weight (kg)	382	2.71	0.46
Retail yield (kg)	249	1.97	0.28
Model, including cold carcass weight (376 kg average cold carcass weight)			
Retail yield (kg)	249	NS	−0.0629

Growth to, and carcass weight and retail yield at, 30 months of age (n = 228 cattle). The slopes are the change in the trait per kilogram change in birthweight or weaning weight.

Abbreviations: NA, not applicable; NS, not significant (*P*>.02).

Adapted from Robinson DL, Cafe LM, Greenwood PL. Developmental programming in cattle: consequences for growth, efficiency, carcass, muscle and beef quality characteristics. J Anim Sci 2013;91:1428–42; with permission.

Postnatal Body and Carcass Composition

The magnitude of developmental programming of postnatal body and carcass composition is greatest when substantial reductions in fetal growth occur as a result of chronically restricted nutrient supply to the fetus. As previously highlighted, maternal nutritional and/or placental compromise of nutrient transfer from the maternal circulation to the fetus is particularly important during later stages of pregnancy.[4] More specific effects of maternal nutrition on the development of the carcass tissues are also evident, although these may be quantitatively more modest and may not result in economically meaningful effects at market weights.[3,4]

Bone, including ossification

Postnatal bone growth may or may not be affected by maternal nutrition in sheep. Femur weight and cortical bone density were reduced at 5 months of age in lambs from ewes nutritionally restricted for 6 weeks before parturition.[47] However, restricted maternal nutrition from day 30 of pregnancy until parturition did not affect bone length or density at 3 months of age.[47] Overnutrition of ewes from day 30 of pregnancy until parturition did not affect postnatal bone growth or density in offspring at 3 months of age[47] or at birth of second filial offspring.[48]

Lambs of low birthweight due to placental restrictions on their prenatal growth had less ash in the whole body than normal lambs at any given empty bodyweight up to 20 kg following ad libitum feeding that resulted in rapid postnatal growth.[38] This suggests that bone lacks the capacity to respond as rapidly as the soft tissues to the postnatal increase in nutrient availability. Despite this, lambs of low birthweight did not differ from their higher birthweight counterparts in absolute or relative bone mineral content at 2.3 years of age.[49]

The amount of bone in carcasses of cattle at 30 months of age following maternal nutrition restriction from about day 80 of pregnancy until parturition was reduced as a result of lower birthweight, resulting in slower postnatal growth (see **Table 4**).[3]

Table 2
Effects of birthweight and weaning weight on feed intake and efficiency

Trait, kg	Mean	Birthweight (Slope/kg Birthweight)	Weaning Weight (Slope/kg Weaning weight)
Feedlot intake (kg DM/d)	12.1	0.09	0.009
Feedlot intake, (kg DM/d): at equivalent liveweight at feedlot entry	12.1	NS	NS
Feed conversion ratio (kg DM/kg gain)	9.4	NS	0.022
Feed conversion ratio (kg DM/kg gain): at equivalent liveweight at feedlot entry	9.4	NS	NS
Residual feed intake (kg DM/d)	0	NS	NS

From 26 to 30 months of age (n = 146 cattle). The slopes are the change in the trait per kilorgam of change in birthweight or weaning weight.
Abbreviation: DM, dry matter.
Adapted from Robinson DL, Cafe LM, Greenwood PL. Developmental programming in cattle: consequences for growth, efficiency, carcass, muscle and beef quality characteristics. J Anim Sci 2013;91:1428–42; with permission.

However, effects of maternal nutrition or birthweight on carcass bone content at an equivalent carcass weight at slaughter were not evident, nor were there any additional effects due to maternal nutrition, beyond those due to birthweight, on the weight of bone in the whole carcass at 30 months of age.[3] Poor maternal nutrition during lactation and lower weaning weight reduced bone content of the carcass at 30 months of age but not at the same carcass weight of 376 kg (**Table 3**).[3]

Ossification score was higher (206 v 195) in low compared with high birthweight cattle at an equivalent carcass weight of 380 kg at 30 months of age,[50] suggesting

Table 3
Effects of birthweight and weaning weight on yield and compositional characteristics

Trait	Mean	Birthweight (Slope/kg Birthweight)	Weaning Weight (Slope/kg Weaning Weight)
Retail yield (kg)	249	1.97	0.28
Fat trim (kg)	55.4	NS	0.10
Bone (kg)	67.6	0.51	0.07
Striploin (kg)	5.97	0.0346	0.0055
Eye round (kg)	2.74	0.0196	0.0015
At equivalent cold carcass weight (376 kg)			
Retail yield (kg)	249	NS	−0.0629
Fat trim (kg)	55.4	NS	0.08
Bone (kg)	67.6	NS	NS
Striploin (kg)	5.97	NS	NS
Eye round (kg)	2.74	NS	−0.001

At 30 months of age (n = 228 cattle). The slopes are the change in the trait per kilogram change in birthweight or weaning weight.
Adapted from Robinson DL, Cafe LM, Greenwood PL. Developmental programming in cattle: consequences for growth, efficiency, carcass, muscle and beef quality characteristics. J Anim Sci 2013;91:1428–42; with permission.

increased bone mineralization as a result of severe fetal growth retardation. However, these effects were not evident within a more comprehensive assessment of factors affecting ossification score (**Table 4**).[3] Effects of maternal nutrition during lactation or of weaning weight on ossification score were not evident (see **Table 4**).[3]

Adipose tissue and fatness

Results of studies on maternal nutritional and intrauterine growth retardation effects on offspring adiposity were comprehensively reviewed.[3,39,51]

In sheep, it can be concluded that prolonged, severe fetal growth retardation resulting in low birthweight, or prolonged and severe maternal nutritional restriction that includes late pregnancy, predisposes offspring to increased fatness during postnatal life. Maternal nutrition before and during early pregnancy to midpregnancy often has little or no effect on body composition at equivalent postnatal liveweight or carcass weights; however, some studies report effects of maternal nutrition during this period on offspring adiposity during postnatal life.[4,39,51] Overfed, obese ewes and control ewes produced offspring similar in liveweight and absolute and relative fat mass at 19.5 months of age. However, when both groups of offspring were then fed ad libitum for 12 weeks, the offspring of the obese ewes became markedly fatter during this period.[52]

Maternal nutritional restriction of grazing cows from day 80 of pregnancy until parturition did not affect rib or rump fat depths (see **Table 4**) or the amount of fat trimmed from the carcass (see **Table 3**) of offspring at 30 months of age or at an equivalent carcass weight of 376 kg.[3] A review of other studies on maternal nutrition of cattle during early pregnancy and/or midpregnancy generally showed small or no effects on carcass fatness.[3] However, midgestational nutrition for 60 days on lower protein

Table 4
Effects of birthweight and weaning weight on carcass characteristics

Trait	Mean	Birthweight (Slope/kg Birthweight)	Weaning Weight (Slope/kg Weaning Weight)
Hot carcass weight (kg)	382	2.71	0.46
Dressing percentage	56.3	ns	NS
Cold side weight (kg)	188	1.33	0.23
Rump fat depth (mm)	20.5	NS	0.039
Rib fat depth (mm)	11.7	NS	NS
Ribeye area (cm²)	89.7	0.52	NS
US marble score	446	NS	NS
Longissimus IMF (%)	6.94	NS	NS
MSA ossification score	200	NS	NS
At equivalent cold carcass weight (376 kg)			
Dressing percentage	56.3	NS	−0.01
Rump fat depth (mm)	20.5	NS	NS
Ribeye area (cm²)	89.7	0.52	NS
MSA ossification score	200	NS	NS

At 30 months of age (n = 228 cattle). The slopes are the change in the trait per kilogram change in birthweight or weaning weight.

Abbreviations: IMF, intramuscular fat; MSA, Meat Standards Australia.

Adapted from Robinson DL, Cafe LM, Greenwood PL. Developmental programming in cattle: consequences for growth, efficiency, carcass, muscle and beef quality characteristics J Anim Sci 2013;91:1428–42; with permission.

native range pasture compared with improved pasture resulted in offspring with similar birthweights but heavier carcasses (348 kg vs 330 kg) with greater rib fat depth at the same age (1.51cm vs 1.11 cm fat depth) and the same carcass weight (1.64 cm vs 1.24 cm fat depth).[53] In comparison with prenatal growth retardation, reduced weaning weight of calves due to poor nutrition of lactating cows was associated with less carcass fat trim and rump fat depth at 30 months of age and less carcass fat trim at the same carcass weight of 376 kg (see **Tables 3** and **4**).[3]

Conflicting results on consequences of maternal nutrition during pregnancy on fatness of offspring can be difficult to reconcile and may result from a range of factors before, during, and after gestation, including prior and subsequent nutrition, and carryover effects on dam lactation performance.[3,4,51]

Yield of meat
Meat yield and muscle characteristics in offspring of cows subjected to a range of maternal nutritional treatments were reviewed by Robinson and colleagues.[3] The findings are consistent with the assertion that, despite effects on growth and development of the fetus, there is considerable plasticity in postnatal systems to regulate skeletal muscle hypertrophy to overcome earlier negative impacts.[4]

Within pasture-based systems, the effects on retail yield at 30 months of age were entirely attributable to differences in size of offspring at this age due to maternal nutrition from day 80 of pregnancy to term, and to birthweight.[3,50] Hence, neither cow nutrition during pregnancy or birthweight influenced meat yield in these offspring at an equivalent carcass weight of 376 kg at 30 months of age (see **Table 3**). In comparison, retail yield increased with increasing weaning weight at 30 months of age but at an equivalent carcass weight (376 kg) declined with increasing weaning weight (see **Table 3**). Various other studies in cattle have assessed the effects of a range of maternal nutritional treatments during midpregnancy and/or late pregnancy on US Department of Agriculture yield grade[54–58] or yield-specific carcass components,[59] with none of the treatments having a significant effect. Similarly, ewe nutrition at 60% of predicted ME requirements from day 45 to 115 of pregnancy had few effects on yield characteristics in sheep.[46]

Reduced birthweight also resulted in all primal cuts in the carcass being smaller at 30 months of age, consistent with difference in growth, size, and retail yield at slaughter; however, there were few effects on a carcass weight–equivalent basis.[60] At 380 kg carcass weight, there was a small difference (1%–2%) in the distribution of retail beef yield between the forequarter and the hindquarter between groups of low and high birthweight calves.[60]

Marbling
Marble score and longissimus muscle intramuscular fat content of cattle at 30 months of age and 376 kg carcass weight were not affected by varying nutrition of cows at pasture from 80 days of pregnancy to term or by birthweight (see **Table 4**).[3] Nor were they affected by cow nutrition during lactation or by weaning weight (see **Table 4**).[3] However, protein supplementation of cows grazing winter range or corn residue systems during late pregnancy increased marbling score irrespective of grazing system.[56] Feeding hay to dams in late pregnancy resulted in offspring with higher marbling score and a tendency toward more intramuscular fat compared with offspring of corn-fed cows.[61] These studies suggest benefits from feeding additional protein, rather than additional energy, to cows during late pregnancy to enhance marbling in offspring.

Eating Quality and Nutritional Attributes of Meat

Influences of maternal nutrition and altered fetal growth on eating quality of meat, if evident, seem to be relatively insignificant compared with later postnatal influences, such as feedlot or pasture finishing, preslaughter management, and abattoir processing. Similarly, prenatal influences on the nutritional attributes of meat, such as fat, protein, and energy content, as a result of changes in carcass composition are generally not significant compared with the influences of genotype and finishing in feedlot compared with pasture.[6] However, the effects of maternal nutrition on more specific aspects of nutrient composition of the meat of their offspring have been little studied in livestock and warrant further investigation.

Within pasture-based rearing and grow-out systems followed by feedlot finishing, maternal nutrition and birthweight had few effects on objective beef quality attributes of offspring, including shear force, compression, cooking loss, ultimate pH, intramuscular fat content, and meat color at 30 months of age (**Table 5**).[3,50] Birthweight explained 2.3% of the variation in striploin color lightness and 1.6% of the variation in eye round (semitendinosus) compression, with no other effects of maternal nutrition or birthweight on meat quality evident. Nutrition of lactating cows at pasture and weaning weight of calves had no effects on objective meat quality attributes (see **Table 5**).[3]

Shear force in the semitendinosus muscle was greater in bull progeny following restriction of dietary protein of cows from 60 day before conception until 24 days postconception, and heat-soluble collagen in the semitendinosus muscle was reduced by the periconceptual nutritional treatment.[62] Other beef quality characteristics in the semitendinosus muscle and the beef quality of the longissimus muscle in these bulls were not affected by the nutritional treatments.[62] Supplementation during

Table 5
Effects of birthweight and weaning weight on beef quality characteristics

Trait	Mean	Birthweight (Slope/kg birthweight)	Weaning Weight (Slope/kg Weaning Weight)
Longissimus lumborum (striploin)			
Shear force (N)	39.7	NS	NS
Compression (N)	14.1	NS	NS
Cooking loss (%)	21.5	NS	NS
Ultimate pH (pH$_u$)	5.48	NS	NS
Color L (lightness)	39.8	0.072	NS
Color a (red-green)	26.5	NS	NS
Color b (yellow-blue)	13.7	NS	NS
Semitendinosus (eye round)			
Shear force (N)	46.1	NS	NS
Compression (N)	22.4	−0.011	NS
Compression (N)	22.4	NS	NS
Cooking loss (%)	21.3	NS	NS

At 30 months of age (n = 228 cattle). The slopes are the change in the trait per kilogram change in birthweight or weaning weight.

Abbreviation: N, Newton.

Adapted from Robinson DL, Cafe LM, Greenwood PL. Developmental programming in cattle: consequences for growth, efficiency, carcass, muscle and beef quality characteristics. J Anim Sci 2013;91:1428–42; with permission.

midpregnancy improved tenderness[53] and, as previously reported, marble score and quality grades of offspring were improved by protein supplementation in late pregnancy.[56] Pregnant cows supplemented with hay during late pregnancy had offspring with improved marbling score and quality grade compared with those of cows supplemented with corn during the same period.[61]

Nutritional restriction during early pregnancy to midpregnancy or late pregnancy did not affect sheep meat quality characteristics at market weights.[46,63–65] More recent evidence suggests periconceptual and late pregnancy maternal fatty acid supplementation may have some limited effects on fatty acid composition in offspring muscle during later life.[66,67]

POSTNATAL AND GENOTYPIC INTERACTIONS WITH MATERNAL NUTRITION AND FETAL DEVELOPMENT DURING PREGNANCY

Studies of interactions between developmental programming of the fetus and factors such as maternal and offspring nutrition from birth to weaning, later life nutritional treatments, and genotype for carcass and meat eating quality characteristics in ruminants have been limited.[3,4,51] There were few interactions between cow nutrition at pasture during pregnancy and from birth to weaning, or between fetal growth to term and subsequent growth to weaning, for growth, efficiency, carcass, yield, and beef quality characteristics to 30 months of age and approximately 380 kg carcass weight.[3] Hence, nutritional effects on offspring during the prenatal and preweaning periods were additive, resulting in exacerbation or amelioration of early life nutritional influences on subsequent productivity. In these studies, there were only a few interactions between sire genotypes for high muscling and high marbling and nutrition and growth of offspring during the fetal and preweaning periods for subsequent beef production, due to consistent effects or lack of effects of the early life treatments on subsequent performance of the offspring in these genotypes (**Boxes 1** and **2**).[3,41,50,60]

CONCLUSIONS

Developmental programming in ruminant livestock has been the subject of increasing attention and study in recent years. There is now an understanding of the magnitude of

---

Box 1
Outcomes of poor cow nutrition at pasture during pregnancy resulting in reduced birthweight

- Slower growth to weaning
- No backgrounding compensation
- Reduced feedlot growth
- Similar feedlot efficiency
- Calves did not catch up in weight
- Little effect on carcass and yield characteristics at equivalent carcass weights
- Little effect on meat quality characteristics
- Virtually no interactions with cow nutrition during lactation or with preweaning growth
- Virtually no interactions with sire genotype

Data from Robinson DL, Cafe LM, Greenwood PL. Developmental programming in cattle: consequences for growth, efficiency, carcass, muscle and beef quality characteristics. J Anim Sci 2013;91:1428–42.

Box 2
Outcomes of poor cow nutrition at pasture during lactation resulting in reduced weaning weight

- Some backgrounding compensation
- Similar feedlot growth and efficiency
- Calves did not catch up in weight
- Little effect on carcass and yield characteristics at equivalent carcass weights
- Little effect on meat quality characteristics
- Additive with prenatal effects
- Virtually no interactions with cow nutrition during pregnancy or with prenatal growth
- Virtually no interactions with sire genotype

Data from Robinson DL, Cafe LM, Greenwood PL. Developmental programming in cattle: consequences for growth, efficiency, carcass, muscle and beef quality characteristics. J Anim Sci 2013;91:1428–42.

---

some of the major early life developmental impacts on meat production in ruminants. Mostly, these effects are mediated by factors that severely affect the growth of the fetus, and may have long-term consequences for growth and size of offspring and, hence, time to reach market weight. Influences of maternal nutritional treatments before and during early pregnancy generally have had only limited impact on meat production in ruminants. Development of nutritional and other treatments to enhance fetal development and postnatal consequences for the productivity of ruminant livestock may be enhanced by molecular methods to characterize epigenetic mediation of altered development. However, the current industry objectives of managing breeding animals to optimize reproductive rates and efficiency to weaning remain pertinent and should result in minimal adverse consequences of developmental programming for growth, efficiency, and meat production of ruminant livestock.

SUMMARY

Maternal regulation of fetal development has long-term consequences for later growth and development of body tissues for meat production. Severely restricted fetal growth in ruminants can reduce postnatal growth capacity, resulting in smaller-for-age animals that take longer to reach market weights but has little effect on feedlot efficiency or carcass and meat quality. Specific nutritional interventions, particularly during later pregnancy, may limit fetal growth retardation and enhance postnatal growth capacity and carcass weight at slaughter, and may improve development of specific tissues such as intramuscular fat. Continued improvements in understanding developmental processes and their regulation will increase the future capacity to improve growth, efficiency, carcasses, and meat quality through developmental programming.

ACKNOWLEDGMENTS

We acknowledge the contribution of the Australian Beef Cooperative Research Centres (Beef CRCs) and it's partner organizations, in particular, the New South Wales Department of Primary Industries (NSW DPI) and Meat & Livestock Australia (MLA), in supporting our Beef CRC research described in this article. We also acknowledge the support of the Department of Animal Science at Cornell University, NSW DPI, and MLA in supporting our sheep research on developmental programming described in this article.

REFERENCES

1. Bell AW, Greenwood PL, Ehrhardt RA. Regulation of metabolism and growth during prenatal life. In: Burrin DJ, Mersmann HJ, editors. Biology and metabolism of growing animals. Amsterdam: Elsevier Science BV; 2005. p. 3–34.
2. Wu G, Bazer FW, Wallace JM, et al. Intrautuerine growth retardation: implications for the animal sciences. J Anim Sci 2006;84:2316–37.
3. Robinson DL, Cafe LM, Greenwood PL. Developmental programming in cattle: consequences for growth, efficiency, carcass, muscle and beef quality characteristics. J Anim Sci 2013;91:1428–42.
4. Bell AW, Greenwood PL. Prenatal origins of postnatal variation in growth, development and productivity of ruminants. Anim Prod Sci 2016;56:1217–32.
5. Sinclair KD, Rutherford KMD, Wallace JM, et al. Epigenetics and developmental programming of welfare and production traits in farm animals. Reprod Fertil Dev 2016;28:1443–78.
6. Greenwood PL, Dunshea FR. Biology and regulation of carcass composition. In: Kerry JP, Ledward D, editors. Improving the sensory and nutritional quality of fresh meat. Cambridge (United Kingdom): Woodhead Publishing; 2009. p. 19–60.
7. Bell AW, Ferrell CL. Freetly HC Pregnancy and fetal metabolism. In: Dijkstra J, Forbes JM, France J, editors. Quantitative aspects of ruminant digestion and metabolism. 2nd edition. Wallingford (United Kingdom): CAB International; 2005. p. 523–50.
8. Greenwood PL, Slepetis RM, Bell AW. Influences on fetal and placental weights during mid to late gestation in prolific ewes well-nourished throughout pregnancy. Reprod Fertil Dev 2000;12:149–56.
9. Altschul M. Early ossification of the fetal ovine skeleton. MSc Thesis. Ithaca (NY): Cornell University; 1987.
10. Hammond J. Physiological factors affecting birth weight. Proc Nutr Soc 1944;2:8–12.
11. Hoffman ML, Reed SA, Pillai SM, et al. The effects of poor maternal nutrition during gestation on offspring postnatal growth and metabolism. J Anim Sci 2017;95: 2222–32.
12. Firth EC, Rogers CW, Vickers M, et al. The bone-muscle ratio of fetal lambs is affected more by maternal nutrition during pregnancy than by maternal size. Am J Physiol 2008;294:R1890–4.
13. Picard B, Lefaucheur L, Berri C, et al. Muscle fibre ontogenesis in farm animal species. Reprod Nutr Dev 2002;42:415–31.
14. Rehfeldt C, Fiedler I, Stickland NC. Number and size of muscle fibres in relation to meat quality. In: te Pas MFW, Everts ME, Haagsman HP, editors. Muscle development in livestock species. Physiology, genetics and meat quality. Wallingford (CT): CABI Publishing; 2004. p. 1–38.
15. Stickland NC, Bayol S, Ashton C, et al. Manipulation of muscle fibre number during prenatal development. In: te Pas MFW, Everts ME, Haagsman HP, editors. Muscle development in livestock species. Physiology, genetics and meat quality. Wallingford (CT): CABI Publishing; 2004. p. 69–82.
16. Oksbjerg N, Therkildsen M. Myogenesis and muscle growth and meat quality. In: Purslow PP, editor. New aspects of meat quality. Duxford (United Kingdom): Woodhead Publishing; 2017. p. 33–62.

17. Greenwood PL, Slepetis RM, Hermanson JW, et al. Intrauterine growth retardation is associated with reduced cell cycle activity, but not myofibre number, in ovine fetal muscle. Reprod Fertil Dev 1999;11:281–91.
18. Du M, Tong J, Zhao J, et al. Fetal programming of skeletal muscle development in ruminant animals. J Anim Sci 2010;88(E Suppl):E51–60.
19. Zhu M-J, Ford SP, Nathanielsz PW, et al. Effect of maternal nutrient restriction in sheep on the development of fetal skeletal muscle. Biol Reprod 2004;71: 1968–73.
20. Greenwood PL, Hunt AS, Hermanson JW, et al. Effects of birth weight and postnatal nutrition on neonatal sheep: II. Skeletal muscle growth and development. J Anim Sci 2000;78:50–61.
21. Alexander G. Quantitative development of adipose tissue in foetal sheep. Aust J Biol Sci 1978;31:489–503.
22. Brameld JM, Greenwood PL, Bell AW. Biological mechanisms of fetal development relating to postnatal growth, efficiency and carcass characteristics in ruminants. In: Greenwood PL, Bell AW, Vercoe PE, et al, editors. Managing the prenatal environment to enhance livestock productivity. Dordrecht (the Netherlands): Springer; 2010. p. 93–119.
23. Du M, Wang B, Xing F, et al. Fetal programming in meat production. Meat Sci 2015;109:40–7.
24. Gemmell RT, Alexander G. Ultrastructural development of adipose tissue in foetal sheep. Aust J Biol Sci 1978;31:505–15.
25. Symonds ME, Pope E, Budge H, et al. The ontogeny of brown adipose tissue. Annu Rev Nutr 2015;35:295–320.
26. Taga H, Chilliard Y, Meunier B, et al. Cellular and molecular large-scale features of fetal adipose tissue: is bovine perirenal adipose tissue brown? J Cell Physiol 2012;227:1688–700.
27. Vernon RG, Robertson JP, Clegg RA, et al. Aspects of adipose-tissue metabolism in foetal lambs. Biochem J 1981;196:819–24.
28. Alexander G, Bennett JW, Gemmell RT. Brown adipose tissue in the new-born calf (Bos taurus). J Physiol 1975;244:223–34.
29. Mitchell AD, Scholz AM, Mersmann HJ. Growth and body composition. In: Pond WG, Mersmann HJ, editors. Biology of the domestic pig. Ithaca (NY): Cornell University Press; 2001. p. 225–308.
30. Gemmell RT, Bell AW, Alexander G. Morphology of adipose cells in lambs at birth and during subsequent transition of brown to white adipose tissue in cold and warm conditions. Am J Anat 1972;133:143–64.
31. Satterfield MC, Dunlap KA, Keisler DH, et al. Arginine nutrition and fetal brown adipose development in nutrient-restricted sheep. Amino Acids 2013;45:489–99.
32. Ojha S, Robinson L, Yazdani M, et al. Brown adipose tissue genes in pericardial adipose tissue of newborn sheep are downregulated by maternal nutrient restriction in late gestation. Pediatr Res 2013;74:246–51.
33. Mühlhäusler BS, Roberts CT, Yuen BSJ, et al. Determinants of fetal leptin synthesis, fat mass, and circulating leptin concentrations in well-nourished ewes in late pregnancy. Endocrinology 2003;144:4947–54.
34. Mühlhäusler BS, Duffield JA, McMillen IC. Increased maternal nutrition increases leptin expression in perirenal and subcutaneous adipose tissue in the postnatal lamb. Endocrinology 2007;148:6157–63.
35. George LA, Uthlaut AB, Long NM, et al. Different levels of overnutrition and weight gain during pregnancy have differential effects on fetal growth and organ development. Reprod Biol Endocrinol 2010;8:75.

36. Long NM, Rule DC, Zhu MJ, et al. Maternal obesity upregulates fatty acid and glucose transporters and increases expression of enzymes mediating fatty acid biosynthesis in fetal adipose tissue depots. J Anim Sci 2012;90:2201–10.

37. Tuersunjiang N, Odhiambo JF, Long NM, et al. (2013) Diet reduction to requirements in obese/overfed ewes from early gestation prevents glucose/insulin dysregulation and returns fetal adiposity and organ development to control levels. Am J Physiol 2013;305:E868–78.

38. Greenwood PL, Hunt AS, Hermanson JW, et al. Effects of birth weight and postnatal nutrition on neonatal sheep: I. Body growth and composition, and some aspects of energetic efficiency. J Anim Sci 1998;76:2354–67.

39. Kenyon PR, Blair HT. Foetal programming in sheep – effects on production. Small Rumin Res 2014;118:16–30.

40. Cafe LM, Hennessy DW, Hearnshaw H, et al. Influences of nutrition during pregnancy and lactation on birth weights and growth to weaning of calves sired by Piedmontese or Wagyu bulls. Anim Prod Sci 2006;46:245–55.

41. Cafe LM, Hennessy DW, Hearnshaw H, et al. Consequences of prenatal and pre-weaning growth for feedlot growth, intake and efficiency of Piedmontese- and Wagyu-sired cattle. Anim Prod Sci 2009;49:461–7.

42. Villette Y, Theriez M. Influence of birth weight on lamb performances. I. Level of feed intake and growth. Ann Zootech 1981;30:151–68.

43. Sibbald AM, Davidson GC. The effect of nutrition during early life on voluntary food intake by lambs between weaning and 2 years of age. Anim Sci 1998;66: 697–703.

44. Geraseev LC, Perez JRO, Carvalho PA, et al. Effects of pre and postnatal feed restriction on growth and production of Santa Ines lambs from weaning to slaughter. Revista Brasilia de Zootecnia 2006;35:237–44.

45. Daniel ZCTR, Brameld JM, Craigon J, et al. Effect of maternal dietary restriction on lamb carcass characteristics and muscle fibre composition. J Anim Sci 2007; 85:1565–76.

46. Piaggio L, Quintans G, San Julian R, et al. Growth, meat and feed efficiency traits of lambs born to ewes submitted to energy restriction during mid gestation. Animal 2018;12:256–64.

47. Pillai SM, Sereda NH, Hoffman ML, et al. Effects of poor maternal nutrition during gestation on bone development and mesenchymal stem cell activity in offspring. PLoS One 2016;1(12):e0168382.

48. Shasa DR, Odhiambo JF, Long NM, et al. Multigenerational impact of maternal overnutrition/obesity in the sheep on the neonatal leptin surge in granddaughters. Int J Obes 2015;39:695–701.

49. Louey S, Cock ML, Harding R. Long term consequences of low birth weight on postnatal growth, adiposity and brain weight at maturity in sheep. J Reprod Dev 2005;51:59–68.

50. Greenwood PL, Cafe LM, Hearnshaw H, et al. Long-term consequences of birth weight and growth to weaning carcass, yield and beef quality characteristics of Piedmontese- and Wagyu-sired cattle. Aust J Exp Agric 2006;46:257–69.

51. Greenwood PL, Bell AW, Vercoe PE, et al, editors. Managing the prenatal environment to enhance livestock productivity. Dordrecht: Springer; 2010. IAEA.

52. Long NM, George LA, Uthlaut AB, et al. Maternal obesity and increased nutrient intake before and during gestation in the ewe results in altered growth, adiposity, and glucose tolerance in adult offspring. J Anim Sci 2010;88:3546–53.

53. Underwood KR, Tong JF, Price PL, et al. Nutrition during mid to late gestation affects growth, adipose tissue deposition, and tenderness in cross-bred beef steers. Meat Sci 2010;86:588–93.
54. Banta JP, Lalman DL, Owens FN, et al. Effects of interval feeding whole sunflower seeds during mid to late gestation on performance of beef cows and their progeny. J Anim Sci 2006;84:2410–7.
55. Stalker LA, Adams DC, Klopfenstein TJ, et al. Effects of pre- and postpartum nutrition on reproduction in spring calving cows and calf feedlot performance. J Anim Sci 2006;84:2582–9.
56. Larson DM, Martin JL, Adams DC, et al. Winter grazing system and supplementation during late gestation influence performance of beef cows and steer progeny. J Anim Sci 2009;87:1147–55.
57. Mohrhauser DA, Taylor AR, Underwood KR, et al. The influence of maternal energy status during midgestation on beef offspring carcass characteristics and meat quality. J Anim Sci 2015;93:786–93.
58. Mulliniks JT, Sawyer JE, Harrelson FW, et al. Effect of late gestation bodyweight change and condition score on progeny feedlot performance. Anim Prod Sci 2016;56:1998–2003.
59. Tudor GD, Utting DW, O'Rourke PK. The effect of pre- and post-natal nutrition on the growth of beef cattle. III The effect of severe restriction in early post-natal life on development of the body components and chemical composition. Aust J Agric Res 1980;31:191–204.
60. Greenwood PL, Cafe LM, Hearnshaw H, et al. Consequences of prenatal and preweaning growth for yield of primal cuts from 30 month-old Piedmontese and Wagyu-sired cattle. Anim Prod Sci 2009;49:468–78.
61. Radunz AE, Fluharty FL, Relling AE, et al. Prepartum dietary energy source fed to beef cows: II. Effects on progeny postnatal growth, glucose tolerance, and carcass composition. J Anim Sci 2012;90:4962–74.
62. Alvarenga TIRC, Copping KJ, Han X, et al. The influence of peri-conception and first trimester dietary restriction of protein in cattle on meat quality traits of entire male progeny. Meat Sci 2016;121:141–7.
63. Tygesen MP, Harrison AP, Therkildsen M. The effect of maternal nutrient restriction during late gestation on muscle, bone and meat parameters in five month old lambs. Livest Sci 2007;110:230–41.
64. Krausgrill DI, Tulloh NM, Shorthose WR, et al. Effects of weight loss in ewes in early pregnancy on muscles and meat quality of lambs. J Agric Sci Camb 1999;132:103–16.
65. Nordby DJ, Field RA, Riley ML, et al. Effects of maternal undernutrition during early pregnancy on growth, muscle cellularity, fiber type and carcass composition in lambs. J Anim Sci 1987;64:1419–27.
66. Hopkins DL, Clayton EH, Lamb TA, et al. The impact of supplementing lambs with algae on growth, meat traits and oxidative status. Meat Sci 2014;98:135–41.
67. Martin ACC, Coleman DN, Garcia LG, et al. Prepartum fatty acid supplementation in sheep III. Effect of eicosapentaenoic acid and docosahexaenoic acid during finishing on performance, hypothalamus gene expression, and muscle fatty acid composition in lambs. J Anim Sci 2018;96:5300–10.

Developmental Programming of Fertility in Livestock

Robert A. Cushman, PhD[a],*, George A. Perry, PhD[b]

KEYWORDS

- Fertility • Developmental programming • Puberty • Gonadal development

KEY POINTS

- "Programming" is generally thought to occur at times when critical events in development occur.
- Developmental programming results in physiologic differences in genetically similar animals owing to modifications of the function of the epigenome.
- Although developmental programming has been studied for its negative impacts on growth and performance, it may be possible to apply developmental programming within production systems to target animals toward their final niche, such as the development of highly fertile replacement females.
- Female fertility is an area of application where we have had some success.
- We have also been able to program the development of the gonads and age at puberty; however, this has not translated to changes in fertility.

INTRODUCTION

Developmental programming has been studied extensively for its role in preventing offspring from expressing their total genetic potential for growth owing to stress and insults suffered during fetal development and early life.[1] This can be influenced by external factors such as environmental stressors and internal factors such as age of the dam, which are believed to permanently alter the epigenome of the target organism. Although developmental programming has been studied for its negative effects, there is evidence of the positive effects of developmental programming on progeny performance in some cases. Studies have demonstrated improved fertility of female progeny in response to fetal programming,[2,3] but the exact mechanisms remain

Disclosure Statement: See last page of article.
a Nutrition and Environmental Management Research Unit, USDA, ARS, US Meat Animal Research Center, State Spur 18D, Clay Center, NE 68933, USA; b Department of Animal Science, South Dakota State University, North Campus Drive, Brookings, SD 57007, USA
* Corresponding author.
E-mail address: bob.cushman@ars.usda.gov

unclear. Other studies reported an influence of developmental programming on indicator traits of fertility, such as age at puberty and gonadal development, but have not demonstrated a change in fertility of the progeny. Therefore, a better understanding of the biological mechanisms of epigenetic programming and gonadal development are required before we will be able to harness developmental programming efficiently to improve fertility in domestic livestock.

TIMECOURSE IN REPRODUCTIVE DEVELOPMENT

Developmental programming is generally thought to occur at times when critical events in development occur. Thus, to fully understand how future reproductive performance could be impacted in utero and before puberty occurs, we need a thorough understanding of the developmental process of the gonads.

The Developing Gonad

Female gonadal development
In most mammalian species, a critical event in gonadal formation is the colonization of the genital ridge by primordial germ cells. Primordial germ cells can be seen in the undifferentiated gonads of the bovine fetus around day 35[4] and in the ovine fetus around day 23[5] (**Table 1**). Primordial germ cells migrate from the caudal end of the primitive streak into the hindgut by morphogenetic movements as the hindgut forms. Movement into the hindgut mesentery toward the genital ridge is by active migration of primordial germ cells.[9] The preceding active migration is thought to be regulated by both haptotactic and chemotactic factors[9] and occurs along a region expressing stem cell factor.[10]

In the female, primordial germ cells migrate to the cortical region of the developing ovary, which is the same area of the ovary in which stem cell factor is locally expressed in the ovine fetal ovary.[10] Proliferation of primordial germ cells seems to be synchronized, although the stage of fetal development at which proliferation begins and is completed varies from species to species.[4,6,7] In bovine ovaries, primordial germ cells

Table 1
Time course of ovarian development for cattle, sheep, and pigs

	Age in Days Postconception		
	Cattle[4]	Sheep[6]	Pigs[7,8]
Conception			
Mesonephros present		20	
Genital ridge present and being colonized by germ cells	35–36	23	18
Gonadal sex differentiation	39	32	27
Germ cell meiosis initiated	75–80	55	40
Maximum number of germ cells in gonad	110	75	50
First follicles formed	90–170	75	60–70
Most germ cells lost by atresia	150	90	100
First growing follicles observed	90–170	100	70
Most germ cells have completed meiosis	150	120	110
First antral follicles observed	250	135	60[a]
Birth	—	—	—

[a] Indicates days postpartum.
Data from Refs.[4,6–8]

increase from around 16,000 at 50 days postconception to around 2,700,000 at 110 days but decrease to around 108,000 over the next 40 days.[4] The preceding decrease in follicle numbers reduces the size of the follicular pool from which the initiation of primordial follicle growth will occur. Follicular formation and development also begins during fetal development. In the bovine fetal ovary, the cortex and medulla can be identified by 40 to 70 days postconception. Oogonia enter meiosis between days 75 and 80, and meiosis continues until around day 150 postconception. In cattle, between days 90 and 170 postconception the cortical cords (ovigerous cords) become disrupted.[11] The surviving oocytes are surrounded by a single layer of flattened pregranulosa cells and become enclosed in a basement membrane to form primordial follicles. The newly formed primordial follicles can be found in the ovarian cortex directly under the surface epithelium and surrounding the entire ovary. The pool of quiescent bovine primordial follicles remains constant (around 133,000 per animal) until the animal is 4 to 6 years old, after which the follicular pool is slowly reduced through atresia and ovulation to close to zero around age 20. There is some evidence that the size of the ovarian reserve may positively influence fertility in cattle.[12,13]

Male gonadal development

Like the development of the ovary in females, primordial germ cells migrate from the caudal end of the primitive streak into the hindgut and colonize the genital ridge during early gestation. Specifically, in the male during the earliest stages of development of the gonad, the rudimentary rete can be observed at a crown rump length of 1 to 2 cm in the ram, boar, and bull.[14–16] By 7 to 10 cm (approximately 10 weeks of gestation for bulls), the interstitial cells begin to appear en masse around the developing seminiferous tubules. Beyond 20 cm in all 3 species, there is an increase in seminiferous tubules and a decrease in interstitial cells as the gonad takes on the morphologic appearance of a testis. Beyond this point, the testes increase in size until spermatogenesis begins around puberty.[17]

FEMALE FERTILITY
Fetal Programming

In beef cattle, it is well-established that heifers that conceive early in their first breeding season produce a greater number of calves.[18,19] Therefore, the objective of developmental programming with respect to female fertility should be to produce replacement heifers that are highly fertile, pubertal by 12 months of age, and, in the absence of hormonal synchronization, able to conceive within the first 28 days of their first breeding season. There is evidence that the nutritional status of the dam can impact daughter fertility in beef cattle. Daughters of dams that were provided a protein supplement during the last trimester of gestation were more likely to conceive during the first 21 days of the first breeding season[3]; however, there was no advantage in attainment of puberty among these heifers. At least 1 study, however, reported no effect of maternal supplementation during late gestation on daughter reproductive performance.[20] A lack of an understanding of the physiologic or epigenetic mechanisms involved makes it difficult to reconcile the inconsistency in response across studies and to consistently apply developmental programming to production systems to improve fertility in replacement heifers.

Other studies examined the potential mechanisms involved when applying developmental programming to cows in the third trimester to improve daughter fertility. Cushman and colleagues[2] were able to increase the percentage of daughters that conceived in the first 21 days of a natural breeding season by increasing total feed to the dams during the third trimester. They observed no difference in age at puberty or the percentage of the heifers that had attained puberty by the start of the first breeding season. In addition, they observed no differences in the number of antral follicles detectable by ultrasound examination at 13.5 months of age. Similarly, using distiller's grains fed to beef heifers during late gestation, Gunn and colleagues[21] were able to increase the percentage of daughters conceiving to artificial insemination with no detectable change in attainment of puberty, number of antral follicles detectable by ultrasound examination at 1 year of age, or overall pregnancy rates.

In a study that examined development of the fetal ovary in cattle, a high plane of maternal nutrition fed to cows during mid to late gestation decreased the number of primordial follicles in the ovaries of female fetuses.[22] This was apparently due to an increase in the rate of activation of primordial follicles in the fetal ovaries because there was a corresponding increase in numbers of growing microscopic preantral and antral follicles. This increase in microscopic antral follicles was either below the sensitivity of detection by ultrasound examination in the previous studies or absent by the time an ultrasound examination was performed on heifers at 1 year of age.[2,21] If activation is truly increased in fetal ovaries of daughters of cows fed a high plane of nutrition during late gestation, this could imply an increased rate of depletion of the ovarian reserve and decreased reproductive lifespan; however, no heifers were retained for ultrasound evaluation of antral follicle numbers at breeding age or to determine the impact of the programming on reproductive performance. These studies clearly demonstrate the limitations of the scope of studies examining developmental programming of the gonad and its relationship to fertility and reproductive longevity.

During early embryonic development, reduced maternal nutrient intake in beef cows decreases embryonic growth and quality (**Table 2**). It seems likely that, during this window of development, perturbations could have long-term impacts on the growth and development of the progeny by altering blastomere number, growth trajectory, and proliferation of primordial germ cells. Daughters of heifers in which nutrient intake was restricted during this developmental window had fewer antral follicles at 1 year of age,[29] but in this study no histologic evaluation of the ovarian reserve was performed and no fertility data were reported.

Among other livestock species, there is relatively little published evidence of fetal programming influencing daughter fertility. In sheep, maternal nutrient restriction during early to mid gestation decreased circulating progesterone concentrations in daughters at 6 years of age.[30] There were, however, no reports that this treatment impacted fertility of the daughters at any age. There is some evidence that the treatment of ewes with testosterone during gestation can cause insulin insensitivity in daughters. The ewe lambs had altered folliculogenesis and a delayed onset of puberty, but, once again, the data demonstrating a negative impact on fertility in these females have not been reported. In pigs, fewer gilts farrowed by gilts that remained in gestation crates throughout gestation reached puberty by 165 days of age than gilts farrowed from gilts that were in pens throughout gestation or from gilts that were in crates for the first 30 days of gestation and then moved to pens.[31] Maternal exercise during gestation increased proliferation in fetal and neonatal ovaries of daughters.[32] The overall conclusion from these data would be that ovarian development is sensitive to stress during gestation in livestock species; however, there is no published evidence that this translates to differences in fertility or reproductive longevity.

Postnatal Developmental Programming

The nutritional programming of heifers during the first year of life can influence the onset of puberty and the size of the ovarian reserve. When beef heifers were fed to attain a high rate of gain between 4 and 6 months of age, the onset of puberty occurred

	Table 2	
Impact of nutrient restriction around fertilization on early bovine embryonic development		
Fetal Age (d)	**Reproductive Event**	**Impact of Nutrient Restriction Around Day 0**
0	Estrus	Tended to increase interval to and decrease estrus expression[23,24]
1	Conception	No effect on fertilization[23,24]
2	First cleavage[25,26]	
3	Eight-cell stage[25]	
4	Maternal to zygotic transition[27]	
5	16–32 cell stage (morula)[25,26]	
7–8	Blastocyst[25,26,28]	Decreased embryo stage and quality[23,24]
8	Expanded blastocyst[25]	
9–11	Hatching[25,26]	
12–13	Elongation[25,26]	
15–17	Maternal recognition of pregnancy[26]	Decreased embryo size
21–22	Adhesion to the endometrium[26]	
23	Binucleate cells appear[26]	
25	Interdigitation at cotyledons[26]	
42	Definitive placentation and organogenesis[26]	Decreased embryo survival[23,24]
Birth/weaning		Decreased birth weight and decreased weaning weights of calves[24] Decreased antral follicle count in heifer calves[29] Tended to increase 5-hmC methylation[24]

Data from Refs.[23–29]

at a younger age than when heifers were fed to attain a low rate of gain during this developmental window.[33,34] Similar results have been observed based on average daily gain from birth to weaning, because heifers with a greater average daily gain between birth and weaning have a younger age at puberty.[2,35] When heifers were restricted early and then fed for a high rate of gain between 6 and 9 months of age, puberty was attained at a greater rate between 12 and 14 months of age.[34,36] This finding is important because it increased the percentage of heifers that attained puberty without increasing the rate of precocious puberty, which may place a heifer in peril of becoming pregnant too young.

In contrast, a model that reduced caloric intake between 8 and 11 months and then increased caloric intake between 11 and 14 months had no influence on attainment of puberty in cross-bred beef heifers.[37,38] Heifers developed in this fashion instead had increased numbers of primordial follicles in their ovaries at the start of their first breeding season, although there was no correlated increase in the numbers of antral follicles. This finding agrees with rodent models that have demonstrated an increase in the size of the ovarian reserve when caloric intake was restricted in the peripubertal period.[39] The most likely mechanism is a slowing of primordial follicle activation when caloric intake is restricted. To date, no data have been published to clearly demonstrate that either of these development methods improves the heifer pregnancy rate or reproductive longevity. Therefore, it cannot be concluded that this is a true developmental programming of fertility.

MALE FERTILITY
Fetal Programming

Developmental programming of male fertility in livestock has been studied less, probably because in production agriculture fewer males are retained as breeding stock. There has, however, been some investigation of fetal programming. Maternal nutritional and hormonal treatments during gestation altered sperm quality, testicular development, and the onset of puberty in bull progeny. Cows provided low protein intake around the time of conception produced male progeny with a delay in attainment of puberty and decreased sperm quality.[40] Similarly, a high plane of maternal nutrition fed to cows in mid to late gestation decreased the diameter and the volumetric density of seminiferous cords in the fetal testes.[22] When cows were administered slow-release melatonin implants from day 180 to day 270 of gestation, scrotal circumference but not testes weight or size was greater in bull progeny at weaning.[41] There was no information on age at puberty in this study, and neither study provided data to demonstrate a difference in fertility in the male progeny. What is apparent from these studies is that the growth and composition of the testes can be influenced during fetal development.

Unless gender-sorted semen is to be used in combination with fetal programming to produce progeny of the desired gender, further research is needed here to understand the potential consequences to the fertility of male progeny. In the absence of control of the gender of the progeny, attempts to improve fertility in female progeny could also impact fertility in the male progeny in either beneficial or detrimental ways.

Postnatal Developmental Programming

Postnatal developmental programming may hasten the onset of puberty in bulls.[17] The critical window seems to be the first 6 months of life, when an increased plane of nutrition results in increased gonadotropin secretion and increased testicular development; however, postthaw motility, the capacity to fertilize oocytes in vitro, and the percentage of live sperm were unaffected, once again calling into question the value of such treatments to improve fertility.

It seems that similar studies in the ram and the boar have not been published. This area is where more research is needed, because, in the absence of sexed semen, this method may be a better alternative than fetal programming for male progeny. Postnatal nutritional programming could be applied only to intact males that were expected to be used as breeding stock and would fit the production systems better than fetal programming.

APPLYING DEVELOPMENTAL PROGRAMMING TO IMPROVE FERTILITY

Will it be possible to apply developmental programming to production systems as a way of targeting livestock toward their role in the system (eg, highly fertile replacement females and breeding males in the case of reproduction/genetic propagation)? This question brings us back to the inconsistencies in the literature across studies. These inconsistencies would imply that either it is not real or that we do not understand enough about the underlying biology to harness developmental programming efficiently. Certainly, the age of the dam influences daughter reproductive performance. Beef heifers born to heifers have fewer antral follicles in their ovaries,[42,43] lower circulating concentrations of anti-Müllerian hormone,[44] and decreased fertility[44] compared with heifers born to mature cows. This is in the absence of nutritional treatments and implies that the response in a study could certainly be different based on the age of the females used in the production system.

The stage of gestation when developmental programming is applied can influence the mechanisms involved. It seems that decreased nutrient intake during early gestation can produce the same result as increased nutrient intake during late gestation in cattle, that is, a decreased numbers of follicles.[22,29] The mechanisms are different, however, because the first slows germ cell proliferation while the latter stimulates primordial follicle activation.

There is an influence of litter size on birth weight in polytocous livestock and, even among cattle, birth weights are reduced in twins in triplets. Selection for increased ovulation rate in cattle increased the numbers of follicles in the ovaries[45,46] while decreasing birth weights.[47] Thus, this negative impact of increased litter size on birth weight does not necessarily inhibit the development of the ovarian reserve in offspring, but realizing that the number of fetuses present in utero will most likely influence the response to developmental programming and understanding how to adjust for that will be an important component of applying developmental programming to production systems.

These studies were performed in different regions throughout the world with different climates, different seasonal variations in day lengths, and different nutrient availabilities. How these factors interact with the epigenome and alter its function and response to external inputs is most likely complex and largely unknown. Only through basic biological studies can we hope to dissect these mechanisms. Additionally, there will be genotype interactions with the environment that influence how the animal's epigenome responds to external stimuli. Some biological types will have more extreme responses to specific external stressors than others. An example would be resistance to heat stress in Bos indicus cattle. These differences could be due to differences in noncoding RNA recognition sites and abundance of methylation sites within the genome of a specific breed or genotype.

The response to developmental programming can differ based on gender of the target organism. In pigs, maternal malnutrition influenced progeny differently based on gender.[48] Females progeny prioritized the growth of brain, liver, lungs, kidneys, and intestines, and deemphasized bone and muscle growth in the face of prenatal malnutrition. Therefore, as stated, depending on the goal of the developmental programming, there may be the need to combine developmental programming with gender-sorted semen or some other technology to control gender of the progeny (eg, gender determination and selection of embryos before transfer).

Finally, the thought that programming can be applied in utero and set for life is short sighted based on the biology. It is clear that epigenetic programming continues to change throughout the lifespan in monozygotic human twins.[49] As discussed, postnatal programming occurs. Therefore, in a production system, unforeseen environmental impactors (eg, blizzards, droughts, etc) could cause epigenetic reprogramming and change the trajectory of females that had been previously programmed as highly fertile breeding females. Given all of this information, it remains interesting that increasing the plane of nutrition to cows in late gestation has resulted in improved daughter fertility in several studies,[2,3] indicating that this may be one window of development where fetal programming could be applied with consistent benefits later in life.

DISCLOSURE STATEMENT

The authors have no relationship with any commercial company that has a direct financial interest in the subject matter. The US Department of Agriculture (USDA) prohibits discrimination in all its programs and activities on the basis of race, color, national origin, age, disability, and where applicable, sex, marital status, familial status, parental status, religion, sexual orientation, genetic information, political beliefs, reprisal, or because all or part of an individual's income is derived from any public assistance program. (Not all prohibited bases apply to all programs.) Persons with disabilities who require alternative means for communication of program information (Braille, large print, audiotape, etc) should contact USDA's TARGET Center at (202) 720-2600 (voice and TDD). To file a complaint of discrimination, write to USDA, Director, Office of Civil Rights, 1400 Independence Avenue, SW, Washington, DC 20250-9410, or call (800) 795-3272 (voice) or (202) 720-6382 (TDD). The USDA is an equal opportunity provider and employer.

REFERENCES

1. Gluckman PD, Liggins GC. Regulation of fetal growth. In: Beard RW, Nathanielsz PW, editors. Fetal physiology and medicine. 2nd edition. London: Butterworths; 1984. p. 511–57.
2. Cushman RA, McNeel AK, Freetly HC. The impact of cow nutrient status during the second and third trimesters on age at puberty, antral follicle count, and fertility of daughters. Livest Sci 2014;162:252–8.
3. Martin JL, Vonnahme KA, Adams DC, et al. Effects of dam nutrition on growth and reproductive performance of heifer calves. J Anim Sci 2007;85(3):841–7.
4. Erickson BH. Development and radio-response of the prenatal bovine ovary. J Reprod Fertil 1966;11(1):97.
5. McNatty KP, Fidler AE, Juengel JL, et al. Growth and paracrine factors regulating follicular formation and cellular function. Mol Cell Endocrinol 2000;163(1–2): 11–20.
6. McNatty KP, Smith P, Hudson NL, et al. Development of the sheep ovary during fetal and early neonatal life and the effect of fecundity genes. J Reprod Fertil Suppl 1995;49:123–35.
7. Black JL, Erickson BH. Oogenesis and ovarian development in the prenatal pig. Anat Rec 1968;161(1):45–55.
8. Oxender WD, Colenbrander B, van dewiel DFM, et al. Ovarian development in fetal and prepubertal pigs. Biol Reprod 1979;21(3):715–21.
9. Donovan PJ. Primordial germ cells. In: Knobil E, Neill JD, editors. Encyclopedia of reproduction, vol. 3. New York: Academic Press; 1999. p. 1064–72.
10. Tisdall DJ, Fidler AE, Smith P, et al. Stem cell factor and c-kit gene expression and protein localization in the sheep ovary during fetal development. J Reprod Fertil 1999;116(2):277.
11. Fortune JE, Yang MY, Allen JJ, et al. Triennial Reproduction Symposium: the ovarian follicular reserve in cattle: what regulates its formation and size? J Anim Sci 2013;91(7):3041–50.
12. Cushman RA, Allan MF, Kuehn LA, et al. Evaluation of antral follicle count and ovarian morphology in crossbred beef cows: investigation of influence of stage of the estrous cycle, age, and birth weight. J Anim Sci 2009;87(6):1971–80.
13. McNeel AK, Cushman RA. Influence of puberty and antral follicle count on calving day in crossbred beef heifers. Theriogenology 2015;84(7):1061–6.

14. Baillie AH. The interstitial cells in the testis of the foetal sheep. Q J Microsc Sci 1960;101:475–80.
15. Allen B. The embryonic development of the ovary and the testis of the mammal. Am J Anat 1904;3:89–146.
16. Bascom F. The interstitial cells of cattle with special reference to their embryonic development and significance. Am J Anat 1923;31:223–60.
17. Kenny DA, Byrne CJ. Review: the effect of nutrition on timing of pubertal onset and subsequent fertility in the bull. Animal 2018;12(s1):s36–44.
18. Perry GA, Cushman R. Effect of age at puberty/conception date on cow longevity. Vet Clin North Am Food Anim Pract 2013;29(3):579–90.
19. Cushman RA, Kill LK, Funston RN, et al. Heifer calving date positively influences calf weaning weights through six parturitions. J Anim Sci 2013;91(9):4486–91.
20. Shoup LM, Ireland FA, Shike DW. Effects of dam prepartum supplement level on performance and reproduction of heifer progeny. Ital J Anim Sci 2017;16(1):75–81.
21. Gunn PJ, Schoonmaker JP, Lemenager RP, et al. Feeding distiller's grains as an energy source to gestating and lactating beef heifers: impact on female progeny growth, puberty attainment, and reproductive processes. J Anim Sci 2015;93(2):746–57.
22. Weller M, Fortes MRS, Marcondes MI, et al. Effect of maternal nutrition and days of gestation on pituitary gland and gonadal gene expression in cattle. J Dairy Sci 2016;99(4):3056–71.
23. Beck EE. Effects of maternal plane of nutrition on early embryonic development and offspring performance. Brookings (SD): Department of Animal Science, South Dakota State University; 2017.
24. Douglas RT, Beck EE, Rich JJJ, et al. Effects of pre- and post-insemination maternal plane of nutrition on estrus and embryo development. J Anim Sci 2018;96(Suppl. 2):260–1.
25. Shea BF. Evaluating the bovine embryo. Theriogenology 1981;15(1):31–42.
26. Peters AR. Embryo mortality in the cow. Anim Breeding Abstr 1996;64:587–98.
27. Telford NA, Watson AJ, Schultz GA. Transition from maternal to embryonic control in early mammalian development: a comparison of several species. Mol Reprod Dev 1990;26(1):90–100.
28. Flechon JE, Renard JP. A scanning electron microscope study of the hatching of bovine blastocysts in vitro. J Reprod Fertil 1978;53(1):9–12.
29. Mossa F, Carter F, Walsh SW, et al. Maternal undernutrition in cows impairs ovarian and cardiovascular systems in their offspring. Biol Reprod 2013;88(4):92.
30. Long NM, Tuersunjiang N, George LA, et al. Maternal nutrient restriction in the ewe from early to midgestation programs reduced steroidogenic enzyme expression and tended to reduce progesterone content of corpora lutea, as well as circulating progesterone in nonpregnant aged female offspring. Reprod Biol Endocrinol 2013;11:34.
31. Estienne MJ, Harper AF. Type of accommodation during gestation affects growth performance and reproductive characteristics of gilt offspring. J Anim Sci 2010;88(1):400–7.
32. Kaminski SL, Grazul-Bilska AT, Harris EK, et al. Impact of maternal physical activity during gestation on porcine fetal, neonatal, and adolescent ovarian development. Domest Anim Endocrinol 2014;48:56–61.
33. Gasser CL, Behlke EJ, Grum DE, et al. Effect of timing of feeding a high-concentrate diet on growth and attainment of puberty in early-weaned heifers. J Anim Sci 2006;84(11):3118–22.

34. Cardoso RC, Alves BR, Prezotto LD, et al. Use of a stair-step compensatory gain nutritional regimen to program the onset of puberty in beef heifers. J Anim Sci 2014;92(7):2942–9.

35. Roberts AJ, Gomes da Silva A, Summers AF, et al. Developmental and reproductive characteristics of beef heifers classified by pubertal status at time of first breeding. J Anim Sci 2017;95(12):5629–36.

36. Amstalden M, Cardoso RC, Alves BR, et al. Reproduction symposium: hypothalamic neuropeptides and the nutritional programming of puberty in heifers. J Anim Sci 2014;92(8):3211–22.

37. Amundson OL, Fountain TH, Larimore EL, et al. Postweaning nutritional programming of ovarian development in beef heifers. J Anim Sci 2015;93(11):5232–9.

38. Freetly HC, Vonnahme KA, McNeel AK, et al. The consequence of level of nutrition on heifer ovarian and mammary development. J Anim Sci 2014;92(12): 5437–43.

39. Wang N, Luo LL, Xu JJ, et al. Obesity accelerates ovarian follicle development and follicle loss in rats. Metabolism 2014;63(1):94–103.

40. Copping KJ, Ruiz-Diaz MD, Rutland CS, et al. Peri-conception and first trimester diet modifies reproductive development in bulls. Reprod Fertil Dev 2018;30(5): 703–20.

41. McCarty KJ, Owen MPT, Hart CG, et al. Effect of chronic melatonin supplementation during mid to late gestation on maternal uterine artery blood flow and subsequent development of male offspring in beef cattle. J Anim Sci 2018;96(12): 5100–11.

42. McNeel AK, Soares EM, Patterson AL, et al. Beef heifers with diminished numbers of antral follicles have decreased uterine protein concentrations. Anim Reprod Sci 2017;179:1–9.

43. Walsh SW, Mossa F, Butler ST, et al. Heritability and impact of environmental effects during pregnancy on antral follicle count in cattle. J Dairy Sci 2014;97(7): 4503–11.

44. Akbarinejad V, Gharagozlou F, Vojgani M, et al. Nulliparous and primiparous cows produce less fertile female offspring with lesser concentration of anti-Mullerian hormone (AMH) as compared with multiparous cows. Anim Reprod Sci 2018; 197:222–30.

45. Cushman RA, Hedgpeth VS, Echternkamp SE, et al. Evaluation of numbers of microscopic and macroscopic follicles in cattle selected for twinning. J Anim Sci 2000;78(6):1564–7.

46. Echternkamp SE, Roberts AJ, Lunstra DD, et al. Ovarian follicular development in cattle selected for twin ovulations and births. J Anim Sci 2004;82(2):459–71.

47. Echternkamp SE, Thallman RM, Cushman RA, et al. Increased calf production in cattle selected for twin ovulations. J Anim Sci 2007;85(12):3239–48.

48. Cogollos L, Garcia-Contreras C, Vazquez-Gomez M, et al. Effects of fetal genotype and sex on developmental response to maternal malnutrition. Reprod Fertil Dev 2017;29(6):1155–68.

49. Fraga MF, Ballestar E, Paz MF, et al. Epigenetic differences arise during the lifetime of monozygotic twins. Proc Natl Acad Sci U S A 2005;102(30):10604–9.

Effects on Animal Health and Immune Function

Reinaldo F. Cooke, PhD

KEYWORDS

- Developmental programming • Offspring immunocompetence • Offspring health
- Prenatal nutrition • Supplementation

KEY POINTS

- Pregnant livestock animals should be in adequate nutritional status to ensure optimal nutrient supply for fetal growth, including development of their immune system.
- Cows with insufficient nutrient intake during gestation produce calves with reduced immunity against diseases, such as scours, respiratory disease, and mastitis.
- Supplementing specific nutrients to pregnant animals in adequate basal nutrition, such as trace minerals and essential fatty acids, appears to enhance offspring health and productivity.
- Research is warranted to promote development of animals with robust immunocompetence, and able to cope with the health challenges associated with livestock production practices.

INTRODUCTION: IMMUNE SYSTEM DURING GESTATION

The concept of developmental programming was established using epidemiologic studies that investigated chronic illnesses in humans, such as coronary heart disease and hypertension.[1,2] Using public health data, these studies evaluated offspring conceived and born during short-term food shortages, including famines resultant from the Nazi occupation of Europe.[1] Scientists reported that food shortages affected offspring development in utero, including weight at birth and early life, resulting in greater incidence of chronic diseases in adult life.[2] Subsequent research demonstrated that many adult diseases take root during gestation,[3] whereas prenatal malnutrition, including undernutrition and overnutrition, are major contributors to adverse developmental programming.[4] Nowadays, these findings serve as a foundation for current human health programs, given the recognized lifetime impacts of gestational nutrition on offspring health.[5]

Optimal health is indispensable for welfare and production efficiency across all livestock species. A robust and well-developed immune system is critical for animals to

Disclosure Statement: The author has nothing to disclose.
Department of Animal Science, Texas A&M University, 2471 TAMU, College Station, TX 77843, USA
E-mail address: reinaldocooke@tamu.edu

endure the multitude of health challenges imposed by current production practices. That includes competence within both innate and adaptive immune systems, and adequate function of neuroendocrine systems that regulate homeostasis.[6] Development of these systems requires a sequential series of carefully timed and coordinated events, beginning early in embryonic/fetal life and continuing through the early postnatal period.[7,8] Accordingly, the impacts of developmental programming on livestock health are important across livestock species for production and welfare reasons and are used as a research model for human and other animal species.[3,9]

Since the early 1900s, livestock has been used as a research model to investigate fetomaternal physiology and developmental biology.[10] Initial experimental evidence of developmental programming was obtained from sheep, including alterations in fetal cerebral blood flow known as brain-sparing.[11] Since then, a considerable body of research has been directed toward defining animal nutrient requirements, including during gestation. However, prenatal malnutrition remains a concern in human health and across livestock systems worldwide.[12,13] During gestation, fetal development is a complex process with different systems being established in different schedules, fueled by maternal nutrient supply via the uterus.[14] Nutrients are partitioned among the developing fetal systems according to a preestablished hierarchy, with systems still not fully functional or essential during gestation having low priority over nutrients.[2] Therefore, the immune system is expected to have less priority over nutrients compared with active systems, such as nervous and circulatory, and its development may be impaired if nutrient supply is limited, resulting in a phenomenon known as intrauterine growth restriction.[15]

PRENATAL MALNUTRITION

Most developmental programming research in livestock has focused on nutrient restriction in pregnant ruminants (**Table 1**).[3] Moreover, attention has been placed on traits relevant to production efficiency and product quality,[14,16] but at a lesser extent in livestock welfare and immunity. However, immune dysfunctions and health challenges have a substantial impact on livestock production systems and their products. As an example, the bovine respiratory disease (BRD) complex is the most common and costly disease of feedlot cattle.[17] Such economical losses include, besides cattle mortality, costs associated with wasted feed resources, purchase of pharmaceuticals, and decreased productive efficiency and carcass quality in morbid cattle.[18] Mastitis is generally considered the most costly disease of dairy cattle, with economical losses resulting from discarded milk, reduced milk yield, risk of antibiotic residues, and culling or death of affected animals.[19] Hence, livestock immunocompetence begins to be defined in utero with direct implications to lifelong animal welfare, productivity, and quality of the final product.

Evidence of development programming effects on cattle immunity was noted nearly 45 years ago. Corah and colleagues[20] fed Hereford primiparous heifers with 100% (C diet) or 65% (R diet) of their estimated energy requirements during the last 100 days of gestation, whereas all heifers received 100% of their requirements upon parturition. The investigators noted that C cows gained 36 kg, whereas R cows lost 6 kg, corroborating the designed differences in nutrient supply between treatment groups. Cows assigned to R gave birth to calves 2 kg lighter, whereas neonatal calf mortality was 10% in R cows and 3% in C cows. These same investigators fed Hereford secundiparous cows with the R diet from day −100 to −30 relative to parturition (day 0), either the R diet or a diet providing 117% of their estimated energy requirement (H) from day −29 to 0, and then 100% of their energy requirements upon parturition. Again, neonatal

Table 1
Summary of research investigating the consequences of prenatal malnutrition on offspring health parameters (mentioned in this article)

Reference	Species	Nutritional Insult	Period of Insult	Health Consequences
Corah et al,[20] 1975	Beef cows	65% energy requirements	Last 100 d of gestation	Increased neonatal mortality
Corah et al,[20] 1975	Beef cows	65% energy requirements	Last 100 d of gestation	Increased neonatal mortality and incidence of scours
Stalker et al,[30] 2006	Beef cows	Body reserve loss	Last trimester of gestation	Increased calf death from birth to weaning
Berry et al,[40] 2008	Dairy cows	Negative energy balance	Most of lactation	Reduced survival to second parity and increased milk somatic cell count
Larson et al,[32] 2009	Beef cows	Body reserve loss	Last trimester of gestation	Increased incidence of BRD and gastrointestinal diseases in the feedlot
Hammer et al,[24] 2011	Ewes	60% energy requirements	Mid and late gestation	Increased efficiency in extracting colostrum nutrients
Gonzalez-Recio et al,[41] 2012	Dairy cows	Negative energy balance	Most of lactation	Lived 16 d shorter and reduced metabolic efficiency
Moriel et al,[31] 2016	Beef cows	70% of energy requirements	Last 40 d of gestation	Impaired humoral and physiologic responses to vaccination against BRD pathogens

mortality was 10% in R cows and 0% in H cows. Incidence of scours was 52% in calves from R cows and 33% in calves from H cows, whereas calf mortality from birth to weaning was 29% and 0%, respectively. In both studies, R cows weaned calves ≥12 kg lighter, but milk production was only impacted in R versus H cows. Other experiments corroborated that prenatal undernutrition predisposes young cattle to neonatal diseases, but associated these outcomes with reduced passive immune transfer from malnourished dams.[21,22] Indeed, Funston and colleagues[23] stated developmental programming effects might have confounded effects on neonatal development due to nutritional impacts on mammary gland and colostrum yield. Nevertheless, Hammer and colleagues[24] compared immunoglobulin transfer and neonatal health of lambs born to dams that received 60%, 100%, or 140% of their nutritional requirements during mid and late gestation. These investigators noted serum immunoglobulin G (IgG) levels were greatest in lambs from ewes receiving 60% of their requirements, suggesting these lambs were programmed to be more efficient in extracting colostrum nutrients and survive greater immune challenges. Colostrum production and quality are known to be reduced in undernourished ewes[25,26]; hence, neonatal immunocompetence is likely influenced by prenatal malnutrition via developmental programming and altered mammary gland physiology.[23]

Adequate passive immunity from colostrum has lifelong health implications in humans and livestock species.[27–29] In turn, prenatal malnutrition may also modulate the development of innate and adaptive immune systems, independent of neonatal passive immunity. Stalker and colleagues[30] evaluated Angus-influenced cows receiving supplemental feed or not during the last trimester of gestation to meet their nutrient requirements. The investigators reported nonsupplemented cows lost body reserves during late gestation, whereas supplemented cows maintained adequate nutritional status. Serum IgG concentrations in calves between 24 and 48 hours after birth were not altered by dam nutritional status, whereas calf survivability from birth to weaning was greater in supplemented cows (98.6 vs 93.5% of calves live at weaning, respectively). These results support the findings from Corah and colleagues,[20] suggesting direct consequences of prenatal malnutrition on offspring health and survival. Moriel and colleagues[31] fed Angus cows with 70% (R diet) or 100% (C diet) of their energy requirements during the last 40 days of gestation, whereas they fed all cows $\geq$100% of their energy requirements upon parturition. Serum IgG concentrations at birth and subsequent health and growth responses were similar between calves born from cows receiving C and R diets. All calves were vaccinated against BRD pathogens 10 days after weaning, and calves from R cows had reduced serum concentrations of cortisol, haptoglobin, and antibody titers against bovine viral diarrhea virus-1 upon vaccination. The investigators concluded that prenatal undernourishment, even if short term, impaired vaccination-induced physiologic responses required for proper immunocompetence against BRD pathogens.

Larson and colleagues[32] evaluated Red Angus × Simmental cows receiving supplemental feed or not during late gestation to meet their nutrient requirements. As designed, body condition scores[33] at parturition were increased by 0.25 points in supplemented cows. The steer progeny from both groups was weaned and managed in a feedlot until slaughter, receiving all immunizations and health management required in commercial feed yards. Incidence of BRD and gastrointestinal diseases in the feedlot was less in steers born from supplemented cows compared with cohorts from unsupplemented dams (1.5% vs 11.5% of morbid cattle, respectively). These outcomes corroborate the findings from Moriel and colleagues,[31] indicating reduced immunocompetence against BRD and other diseases in offspring born from cows with inadequate prenatal nutrition. Funston and colleagues[23] proposed additional evidence of developmental programming impacts immunity against BRD. Undernourished cows are known to produce offspring with permanent alterations in their blood pressure.[34,35] In turn, increased fetal blood pressure and resultant myocardial hypertrophy impairs lung vascularization during gestation.[36] Therefore, inadequate lung development may contribute to increased susceptibility of offspring from undernourished gestating cows to develop BRD later in life. Funston and colleagues[23] also noted decreased feedlot performance attributed to adverse developmental programming, including growth efficiency and carcass quality, might result from impaired offspring immunocompetence.

Researchers also investigated developmental programming and immune function in dairy cattle, but at a lesser extent than beef cattle and other ruminants.[37] Nevertheless, dairy cattle are unique models for developmental programming research. Calves are typically removed from dams immediately after birth and offered a common source of colostrum, milk, and/or replacer,[38] reducing the confounding effects of developmental programming and altered mammary gland physiology.[23] In turn, nutritional status during gestation is mostly determined by cow milk yield; high-producing cows are typically in negative nutritional status during most of the pregnancy.[39] Berry and colleagues[40] compiled records from the Irish Cattle Breeding Federation database and analyzed offspring health and productive responses according to dam milk yield during gestation. The investigators reported that increased dam milk yield was associated with reduced progeny milk yield and survival to second parity, in addition to increased milk somatic cell count suggestive of subclinical mastitis.[19] Similar productive implications were noted by Gonzalez-Recio and colleagues,[41] who reported offspring born to dams lactating while pregnant produced 52 kg less milk, lived 16 days shorter, and were metabolically less efficient than cohorts whose fetal life were developed in the absence of maternal lactation. Moreover, negative programming outcomes noted by Gonzalez-Recio and colleagues[41] were increased according to dam milk productivity, precluding the offspring born to the most productive cows to fully express their genetic merit during their adult life. Nevertheless, research investigating the impacts of developmental programming on immunocompetence and health of dairy cattle is still limited, and future efforts should incorporate other diseases relevant to the dairy industry, such as metabolic and reproductive syndromes.[42]

STRATEGIC SUPPLEMENTATION DURING PREGNANCY

Adequate supply of nutrients to pregnant animals is critical to prevent lifelong health implications to offspring (**Table 2**).[23] In turn, providing nutrients beyond requirements during gestation, also known as nutrient flushing,[43] may benefit developmental programming by increasing nutrient delivery to the fetus.[15] Nutrient flushing, however, should not result in metabolic disorders, such as diabetes or obesity, to prevent adverse developmental programming.[3] As an example, pregnant women with normal pregravid weight are recommended to gain 11 to 16 kg during gestation, being 0.42 kg per week during the second and third trimesters.[44] Moreover, 30% of this weight gain should be in body fat reserves to ensure maternal requirements are met and nutrient supply to the fetus is optimal.[44,45] Similarly, Marques and colleagues[46] recommended pregnant cows should become pregnant at an adequate body condition score and moderately gain body reserves during gestation to optimize offspring health and productivity.

Supplementing specific nutrients above requirements during gestation, but below levels that may result in adverse effects, is common in humans and livestock species. As an example, trace minerals are essential for fetal development,[47] given the fetus depends completely on the dam for proper supply of these elements.[48] Zinc (Zn), copper (Cu), manganese (Mn), and cobalt (Co) are required for adequate development of the fetal nervous, reproductive, and immune systems.[47,49] Accordingly, pregnant women often consume supplemental Cu and Zn, despite their requirements for these elements often being met by their basal diet.[50] Following this same rationale, Marques and colleagues[51] supplemented pregnant cows with sulfate sources of Cu, Co, Mn, and Zn (INR diet), or an organic-complexed source of these trace minerals (ORG diet) during the last trimester of gestation. Cows from both supplement groups received the same daily amount of Cu, Co, Mn, and Zn, whereas a group of nonsupplemented cows (CON diet) was also included in the experiment. The basal diet offered to all cows met their requirements for energy, protein, macrominerals, trace minerals, and vitamins. After parturition, cows and calves were managed similarly, receiving a common mineral supplement containing sulfate sources of Cu, Co, Mn, and Zn. The investigators reported the INR and ORG diets increased liver concentrations of Co, Cu, and Zn in cows. Upon calving, Co concentrations in placental cotyledons and newborn calf liver were also greater in both INR and ORG cows compared with CON. However, Cu concentrations in placental cotyledons and Cu and Zn in the newborn calf liver were only increased in ORG compared with CON cows. At weaning, calves from CON cows were 11 kg lighter than calves from INR cows, and 24 kg lighter than calves from ORG cows, and this difference was maintained until slaughter. In

Table 2
Summary of research investigating the impacts of strategic prenatal supplementation on offspring health parameters (mentioned in this article)

Reference	Species	Nutrient Supplemented	Period of Insult	Health Consequences
Lammoglia et al,[60,61] 1999	Beef cows	ω-6 FA	Last 2 mo of gestation	Enhanced cold tolerance by improving storage and thermogenic capacity of brown adipose tissue
Rooke et al,[71] 2001	Swine	ω-3 FA	Throughout gestation	Increased piglet vitality
Encinias et al,[62] 2004	Ewes	ω-6 FA	Last 50 d of gestation	Reduced survival to second parity and increased milk somatic cell count
Garcia et al,[63] 2014	Dairy cows	ω-6 FA	Last 2 mo of gestation	Altered colostrum FA profile
Marques et al,[51] 2016	Beef cows	Co, Cu, Mn, and Zn	Last trimester of gestation	Reduced BRD incidence in the feedlot
Marques et al,[66] 2017	Beef cows	ω-3 and ω-6 FA	Last trimester of gestation	Increased immune-modulated development of muscle cells and intramuscular fatty acid accumulation

terms of health responses, plasma cortisol concentrations after weaning and vaccination were greater in calves from ORG and INR cows, corroborating that dam nutrition impacted offspring neuroendocrine responses elicited by stress stimuli.[31] More importantly, incidence of BRD during feedlot receiving was less in calves from ORG cows (20%) compared with calves from INR (59.1%) and CON cows (42.3%). Collectively, results from Marques and colleagues[51] indicated trace mineral supplementation to late-gestating cows, particularly from organic-complexed sources, had developmental programming implications on offspring growth and immunocompetence.

In humans and livestock species, ω-3 and ω-6 fatty acids (FA) are essential components of cell structure and integrity and play critical roles in several body functions.[52] However, ω-3 and ω-6 FA, such as linoleic and linolenic acids, cannot be synthesized by the body and must be consumed through the diet.[53] During gestation, ω-3 and ω-6 FA supply to the fetus is transferred via the placenta from the dam circulation.[54,55] Both ω-3 and ω-6 FA also have key immunomodulatory roles. Linolenic acid and its ω-3 derivatives are precursors of eicosanoids that results in anti-inflammatory and immunosuppressive compounds, whereas linoleic acid and its ω-6 derivatives are precursors of proinflammatory reactions.[52] In humans, supplementing pregnant women with ω-3 and ω-6 FA is considered critical for optimal fetal and early-life child development, including growth, nervous, and immune responses.[56] As examples, children born from women supplemented with ω-3 FA during pregnancy had increased resistance to allergies and asthma.[57,58] Comparable benefits were reported in swine by Tanghe and De Smet,[59] as supplementing pregnant sows with ω-3 FA improved piglet vitality as well as preweaning and postweaning growth. Supplementing ω-6 FA to pregnant livestock animals enhanced cold tolerance in beef cattle[60,61] and sheep,[62] mainly by improving storage and thermogenic capacity of brown adipose tissue. In fact, Encinias and colleagues[62] reported reduced mortality via starvation and pneumonia in lambs from ewes supplemented with ω-6 FA during gestation.

Nevertheless, these latter outcomes were mostly attributed to supplemental fat, rather than specific FA, on accretion of brown adipose tissue during fetal development.[60–62]

More recently, Garcia and colleagues[63] supplemented pregnant dairy cows with ω-6 FA, via calcium (Ca) salts to prevent extensive ruminal biohydrogenation,[64] during the last 2 months of gestation. The investigators reported ω-6 FA supplementation altered colostrum FA profile, without improving IgG concentrations in colostrum or calf serum. Subsequently, Garcia and colleagues[65] also failed to demonstrate improved immunocompetence in calves born from dairy cows supplemented with Ca salts of ω-6 FA during gestation. Marques and colleagues[66] supplemented pregnant cows with Ca salts of ω-3 and ω-6 FA (SUPP treatment), or an isolipidic supplement based on Ca salts of palmitic and oleic acids (CON treatment). The investigators reported SUPP cows had increased plasma concentrations of ω-3 and ω-6 FA at calving. Offspring growth from birth to feedlot entry (45 days after weaning at 7 months of age) was not impacted by the SUPP treatment nor the incidence of BRD during feedlot receiving (38.3 vs 31.8% for CON and SUPP). Nevertheless, body weight gain in the feedlot was increased by 100 g/d in calves from SUPP cows, resulting in carcasses with greater marbling compared with calves from CON cohorts (539 vs 489 marbling score, respectively). The investigators mentioned that ω-3 and ω-6 FA modulate muscle and adipocyte function in developing tissues via immunomodulatory effects. More specifically, ω-3 FA positively regulate the expression of genes associated with muscle development and function, but reduce expression of genes regulating lipogenesis and intramuscular FA accumulation to favor metabolism of muscle cells.[67] Contrariwise, ω-6 FA have adipogenic effects by increasing the expression of proinflammatory genes in muscle tissues, promoting adipocyte differentiation and marbling in cattle.[68,69] By supplementing ω-3 and ω-6 FA during late gestation, Marques and colleagues[66] suggested accumulation of these FA into fetal tissues was increased, enhancing development of muscle and adipose cells via immune-related mechanisms, translating into increased carcass growth and intramuscular fat accretion when offspring were provided high-energy anabolic feedlot diets.[70]

SUMMARY

Research presented here corroborates the role of developmental programming on life-long offspring health, with direct impacts on their welfare and productive efficiency. In humans and across livestock species, dams should be in adequate nutritional status to ensure optimal supply of nutrients for fetal growth, including maturation of their immune system.[2] Studies in beef and dairy cattle provided evidence that cows with insufficient nutrient intake during gestation generate calves with reduced immunity against diseases, such as scours, BRD, and mastitis.[20,32,40] This outcome seems independent of prenatal nutrition impacts on mammary gland physiology and passive immunity via colostrum.[30,31] In turn, strategic supplementation programs may further stimulate developmental programming in pregnant livestock animals in adequate nutrition status. More specifically, dams should moderately gain body reserves during gestation to ensure nutrient supply to the fetus is optimal.[46] Supplementing specific nutrients, such as trace minerals and essential FA, appear to enhance fetal development and subsequent offspring health and productivity.[51,66] Nevertheless, the specific impacts of developmental programming on livestock immunity are still not fully understood. Research is warranted to promote development of animals with robust immunocompetence and capable of coping with the health challenges of livestock production practices and demands.[3]

REFERENCES

1. Barker DJ. The origins of the developmental origins theory. J Intern Med 2007; 261:412–7.
2. Barker DJ. Developmental origins of chronic disease. Public Health 2012;126: 185–9.
3. Chavatte-Palmer P, Richard C, Peugnet P, et al. The developmental origins of health and disease: importance for animal production. Anim Reprod 2015;12: 505–20.
4. Velazquez MA, Fleming TP. Maternal diet, oocyte nutrition and metabolism and offspring health. In: Coticchio G, Albertini DF, De Santis L, editors. Oogenesis. New York: Springer; 2013. p. 329–51.
5. Barker DJ, Barker M, Fleming T, et al. Support mothers to secure future public health. Nature 2013;504:209–11.
6. Cooke RF. Nutritional and management considerations for beef cattle experiencing stress-induced inflammation. Prof Anim Sci 2017;33:1–11.
7. Holsapple MP, West LJ, Landreth KS. Species comparison of anatomical and functional immune system development. Birth Defects Res B Dev Reprod Toxicol 2003;68:321–34.
8. Bell AW, Greenwood PL, Ehrhardt RA. Regulation of metabolism and growth during prenatal growth. In: Burrin DG, Mersmann HJ, editors. Biology of metabolism in growing animals. Edinburgh (United Kingdom): Elsevier Limited; 2005. p. 7–31.
9. Zinn SA, Govoni KE, Vonnahme KA. Developmental programming: what mom eats matters! Anim Front 2017;7:3–4.
10. Huggett AS. Foetal blood-gas tensions and gas transfusion through the placenta of the goat. J Physiol 1927;62:373–84.
11. Purves MJ, James IM. Observations on the control of cerebral blood flow in the sheep fetus and newborn lamb. Circ Res 1969;25:651–67.
12. Wu G, Bazer FW, Cudd TA, et al. Maternal nutrition and fetal development. J Nutr 2004;134:2169–72.
13. Reed SA, Govoni KE. How mom's diet affects offspring growth and health through modified stem cell function. Anim Front 2017;7:25–31.
14. Du M, Tong J, Zhao J, et al. Fetal programming of skeletal muscle development in ruminant animals. J Anim Sci 2010;88:E51–60.
15. Wu G, Bazer FW, Wallace JM, et al. Intrauterine growth retardation: implications for the animal sciences. J Anim Sci 2006;84:2316–37.
16. Reynolds LP, Caton JS. Role of the pre- and post-natal environment in developmental programming of health and productivity. Mol Cell Endocrinol 2012;354: 54–9.
17. Wolfger B, Timsit E, White BJ, et al. A systematic review of bovine respiratory disease diagnosis focused on diagnostic confirmation, early detection, and prediction of unfavorable outcomes in feedlot cattle. Vet Clin North Am Food Anim Pract 2015;31:351–65.
18. Griffin D. The monster we don't see: Subclinical BRD in beef cattle. Anim Health Res Rev 2014;15:138–41.
19. Ruegg PL. Investigation of mastitis problems on farms. Vet Clin North Am Food Anim Pract 2003;19:47–73.
20. Corah LR, Dunn TG, Kaltenbach CC. Influence of prepartum nutrition on the reproductive performance of beef females and the performance of their progeny. J Anim Sci 1975;41:819–24.

21. Hough RL, McCarthy FD, Kent HD, et al. Influence of nutritional restriction during late gestation on production measures and passive immunity in beef cattle. J Anim Sci 1990;68:2622–7.

22. Quigley JD, Drewry JJ. Nutrient and immunity transfer from cow to calf pre- and postcalving. J Dairy Sci 1998;81:2779–90.

23. Funston RN, Larson DM, Vonnahme KA. Effects of maternal nutrition on conceptus growth and offspring performance: implications for beef cattle production. J Anim Sci 2010;88:E205–15.

24. Hammer CJ, Thorson JF, Meyer AM, et al. Effects of maternal selenium supply and plane of nutrition during gestation on passive transfer of immunity and health in neonatal lambs. J Anim Sci 2011;89:3690–8.

25. Swanson TJ, Hammer CJ, Luther JS, et al. Effects of plane of nutrition and selenium supplementation on colostrum quality and mammary development in pregnant ewe lambs. J Anim Sci 2008;86:2415–23.

26. Mulder R, Fosgate GT, Tshuma T, et al. The effect of cow-level factors on colostrum quality, passive immunity and health of neonatal calves in a pasture-based dairy operation. Anim Prod Sci 2018;58:1225–32.

27. Wittum TE, Perino LJ. Passive immune status at postpartum hour 24 and long-term health and performance of calves. Am J Vet Res 1995;56:1149–54.

28. Weaver DM, Tyler JW, VanMetre DC, et al. Passive transfer of colostral immunoglobulins in calves. J Vet Intern Med 2000;14:569–77.

29. Victora CG, Bahl R, Barros AJ, et al. Breastfeeding in the 21st century: epidemiology, mechanisms, and lifelong effect. Lancet 2016;387:475–90.

30. Stalker LA, Adams DC, Klopfenstein TJ, et al. Effects of pre- and postpartum nutrition on reproduction in spring calving cows and calf feedlot performance. J Anim Sci 2006;84:2582–9.

31. Moriel P, Piccolo MB, Artioli LFA, et al. Short-term energy restriction during late gestation of beef cows decreases post-weaning calf humoral immune response to vaccination. J Anim Sci 2016;94:2542–52.

32. Larson DM, Martin JL, Adams DC, et al. Winter grazing system and supplementation during late gestation influence performance of beef cows and steer progeny. J Anim Sci 2009;87:1147–55.

33. Wagner JJ, Lusby KS, Oltjen JW, et al. Carcass composition in mature Hereford cows: Estimation and effect on daily metabolizable energy requirement during winter. J Anim Sci 1988;66:603–12.

34. Langley SC, Jackson AA. Increased systolic blood pressure in adult rats induced by fetal exposure to maternal low protein diets. Clin Sci 1994;86:217–22.

35. Murotsuki J, Challis JRG, Han VKM, et al. Chronic fetal placental embolization and hypoxaemia cause hypertension and myocardial hypertrophy in fetal sheep. Am J Phys 1997;272:R201–7.

36. Fabris VE, Pato MD. Progressive lung and cardiac changes associated with pulmonary hypertension in the fetal rat. Pediatr Pulmonol 2001;31:344–53.

37. Roche JR, Friggens NC, Kay JK, et al. Invited review: body condition score and its association with dairy cow productivity, health, and welfare. J Dairy Sci 2009;92:5769–801.

38. Godden S. Colostrum management for dairy calves. Vet Clin North Am Food Anim Pract 2008;24:19–39.

39. Lucy MC. Reproductive loss in high-producing dairy cattle: where will it end? J Dairy Sci 2001;84:1277–93.

40. Berry DP, Lonergan P, Butler ST, et al. Negative influence of high maternal milk production before and after conception on offspring survival and milk production in dairy cattle. J Dairy Sci 2008;91:329–37.
41. Gonzalez-Recio O, Ugarte E, Bach A. Trans-generational effect of maternal lactation during pregnancy: a Holstein cow model. PLoS One 2012;7:e51816.
42. Opsomer G, Van Eetvelde M, Kamal M, et al. Epidemiological evidence for metabolic programming in dairy cattle. Reprod Fertil Dev 2017;29:52–7.
43. Dunn TG, Moss GE. Effects of nutrient deficiencies and excesses on reproductive efficiency of livestock. J Anim Sci 1992;70:1580–93.
44. National Research Council. Weight gain during pregnancy: reexamining the guidelines. Washington, DC: National Academies Press; 2010.
45. Lederman SA, Paxton A, Heymsfield SB, et al. Body fat and water changes during pregnancy in women with different body weight and weight gain. Obstet Gynecol 1997;90:483–8.
46. Marques RS, Cooke RF, Rodrigues MC, et al. Impacts of cow body condition score during gestation on weaning performance of the offspring. Livest Sci 2016;191:174–8.
47. Hostetler CE, Kincaid RL, Mirando MA. The role of essential trace elements in embryonic and fetal development in livestock. Vet J 2003;166:125–39.
48. Hidiroglou M, Knipfel JE. Maternal fetal relationships of copper, manganese and sulfur in ruminants. A review. J Dairy Sci 1981;64:1637–47.
49. Pepper MR, Black MM. B12 in fetal development. Semin Cell Dev Biol 2012;22:619–23.
50. Ladipo OA. Nutrition in pregnancy: mineral and vitamin supplements. Am J Clin Nutr 2000;72:280S–90S.
51. Marques RS, Cooke RF, Rodrigues MC, et al. Effects of organic or inorganic Co, Cu, Mn, and Zn supplementation to late-gestating beef cows on productive and physiological responses of the offspring. J Anim Sci 2016;94:1215–26.
52. Schmitz G, Ecker J. The opposing effects of n-3 and n-6 fatty acids. Prog Lipid Res 2008;47:147–55.
53. Hess BW, Moss GE, Rule DC. A decade of developments in the area of fat supplementation research with beef cattle and sheep. J Anim Sci 2008;86:E188–204.
54. Noble RC, Shand JH, Drummond JT, et al. "Protected" polyunsaturated fatty acid in the diet of the ewe and the essential fatty acid status of the neonatal lamb. J Nutr 1978;108:1868–76.
55. Innis SM. Essential fatty acid transfer and fetal development. Placenta 2005;26:S70–5.
56. Greenberg JA, Bell SJ, Van Ausdal W. Omega-3 fatty acid supplementation during pregnancy. Rev Obstet Gynecol 2008;1:162–9.
57. Krauss-Etschmann S, Hartl D, Rzehak P, et al. Decreased cord blood IL-4, IL-13, and CCR4 and increased TGF-beta levels after fish oil supplementation of pregnant women. J Allergy Clin Immunol 2008;121:464–70.
58. Olsen SF, Østerdal ML, Salvig JD, et al. Fish oil intake compared with olive oil intake in late pregnancy and asthma in the offspring: 16 y of registry-based follow-up from a randomized controlled trial. Am J Clin Nutr 2008;88:167–75.
59. Tanghe S, De Smet S. Does sow reproduction and piglet performance benefit from the addition of n-3 polyunsaturated fatty acids to the maternal diet? Vet J 2013;197:560–9.
60. Lammoglia MA, Bellows RA, Grings EE, et al. Effects of prepartum supplementary fat and muscle hypertrophy genotype on cold tolerance in newborn calves. J Anim Sci 1999;77:2227–33.

61. Lammoglia MA, Bellows RA, Grings EE, et al. Effects of feeding beef females supplemental fat during gestation on cold tolerance in newborn calves. J Anim Sci 1999;77:824–34.
62. Encinias HB, Lardy GP, Encinias AM, et al. High linoleic acid safflower seed supplementation for gestating ewes: effects on ewe performance, lamb survival, and brown fat stores. J Anim Sci 2004;82:3654–61.
63. Garcia M, Greco LF, Favoreto MG, et al. Effect of supplementing fat to pregnant nonlactating cows on colostral fatty acid profile and passive immunity of the newborn calf. J Dairy Sci 2014;97:392–405.
64. Sukhija PS, Palmquist DL. Dissociation of calcium soaps of long-chain fatty acids in rumen fluid. J Dairy Sci 1990;73:1784–7.
65. Garcia M, Greco LF, Favoreto MG, et al. Effect of supplementing essential fatty acids to pregnant nonlactating Holstein cows and their preweaned calves on calf performance, immune response, and health. J Dairy Sci 2014;97:5045–64.
66. Marques RS, Cooke RF, Rodrigues MC, et al. Effects of supplementing calcium salts of polyunsaturated fatty acids to late-gestating beef cows on performance and physiological responses of the offspring. J Anim Sci 2017;95:5347–57.
67. Hiller B, Hocquette JF, Cassar-Malek I, et al. Dietary n-3 PUFA affect lipid metabolism and tissue function-related genes in bovine muscle. Br J Nutr 2012;108: 858–63.
68. Moriel P, Johnson SE, Vendramini JMB, et al. Effects of calf weaning age and subsequent management systems on growth performance and carcass characteristics of beef steers. J Anim Sci 2014;92:3598–609.
69. Mangrum KS, Tuttle G, Duckett SK, et al. The effect of supplementing rumen undegradable unsaturated fatty acids on marbling in early-weaned steers. J Anim Sci 2016;94:833–44.
70. Harper GS, Pethick DW. How might marbling begin? Aust J Exp Agric 2004;44: 653–62.
71. Rooke JA, Sinclair AG, Edwards SA. Feeding tuna oil to the sow at different times during pregnancy has different effects on piglet long-chain polyunsaturated fatty acid composition at birth and subsequent growth. Br J Nutr 2001;86:21–30.

In Utero Heat Stress Programs Reduced Performance and Health in Calves

Geoffrey E. Dahl, PhD*, Amy L. Skibiel, PhD, Jimena Laporta, PhD

KEYWORDS

- Mammary development • Methylation • Milk yield • Heat stress

KEY POINTS

- In utero heat stress reduces the birth weight of calves.
- In utero heat stress compromises passive transfer.
- Methylation patterns differ in hepatic and mammary tissues after in utero heat stress.
- Compared with calves born to cooled dams, calves from heat stressed dams have lower milk yields.

INTRODUCTION: EFFECTS OF LATE GESTATION HEAT STRESS ON THE DAM

It is well-recognized that heat stress, characterized by high ambient temperature and relative humidity, is a major factor adversely affecting cattle throughout the world, even in temperate regions.[1] Heat stressed dairy cows are more vulnerable to disease, have reduced fertility, and drastically lower milk production.[2] In fact, milk yield decreases of up to 40% have been reported,[1,3,4] which is partially attributed to the reduced feed intake of heat stressed cows, with the remaining decline caused by physiologic adjustments in an effort to dissipate metabolic heat.[5,6] It is estimated that, in the United States alone, environmental heat stress on lactating cows costs the dairy industry more than $1.5 billion in losses annually owing to decreased milk yield and increased morbidity and mortality.[1,7] For that reason, many farms in the United States have adopted heat abatement systems, such as fans and water sprayers, to actively cool lactating cows.[8] However, this estimation only accounts for lactating cows. Our recent study estimated that heat stress

Disclosure Statement: Work reported in this paper was supported by grants from the National Science Foundation (Award #1247362 to GED), USDA-NIFA (Award #2015–67015–23409 to GED) and the UF/IFAS Climate Change Grant Program (to JL).
Department of Animal Sciences, Institute of Food and Agricultural Sciences, University of Florida, Gainesville, 2250 Shealy Drive, POB 110910, FL 32611, USA
* Corresponding author.
E-mail address: gdahl@ufl.edu

occurring only during the dry period translates into an additional $810 million in milk losses annually.[9] Dairy industries in hot states such as Florida, Texas, and California suffer the greatest economic impact, but even states such as Michigan and Wisconsin experience hundreds of kilograms of milk losses in a typical lactation owing to dry period heat stress.

Although cows are highly susceptible to heat stress during lactation, heat stress during the dry period, the nonlactating period between successive lactations, also negatively impacts milk production in the subsequent lactation.[10–12] For example, housing late gestation dry cows (from approximately 230 days pregnant to calving) in shaded barns without access to active cooling devices, such as water soakers and fans, induces heat stress that cause systemic and tissue-specific changes that culminate in milk loss (approximately 5 kg per cow per day) in the subsequent lactation.[10,12–14] Moreover, when cows are heat stressed during the dry period, they exhibit altered mammary gland microstructure during early subsequent lactation, featuring fewer alveoli compared with cooled cows.[15] Also, nonlactating, heat-stressed cows have aberrant patterns of hepatic protein expression consistent with oxidative stress, mitochondrial dysfunction, and liver-specific changes in lipid and glucose metabolism early postpartum.[16]

Heat stress, therefore, negatively impacts mature cows during established lactation and during the dry period, wherein it causes recoverable effects on mammary output and metabolic accommodations to reduce heat load. In dry cows, heat stress programs mammary growth and reduces yield in the subsequent lactation. The reduction in yield is associated with decreased autophagy[17] and apoptosis[11] during involution shortly after cessation of milk removal, followed by a delay in epithelial cell proliferation later in the dry period.[11] These programming effects, however, seem to be transient and restricted to that lactation, whereas the impacts of in utero heat stress on the developing fetus are permanent and transgenerational. Those effects are the focus of the remainder of this article.

DEVELOPMENTAL PROGRAMMING AND THE MAMMARY GLAND

During specific developmental windows, conditions experienced in early life can affect gene expression, cells, tissues, and organs with consequences for future physiologic function, health, and disease outcomes later in life,[18,19] a concept known as developmental programming.[20] The dry period of a dairy cow coincides with the last trimester of gestation, a time of maximal fetal development.[21] As a cow is stressed in late gestation, so too is the fetus, which shapes their future performance. It is evident from nutritional studies in ruminants that conditions experienced early in life can program future mammary function. Fetuses of ewes fed a maintenance diet throughout gestation have heavier mammary glands compared with fetuses carried by ewes on an ad libitum diet. Independent of diet, ewe size during pregnancy also influences fetal mammary development. Fetuses of heavier ewes have a larger mammary ductal area.[22] Further, lambs of heavier ewes and those fed a maintenance diet also produce more milk during their first lactation, indicative of in utero programming of mammary function through changes in early gland development.

Early life nutritional manipulation can also impact mammary development. Calves fed a higher plane of nutrition during the preweaning period produce more milk during the first lactation.[23,24] This may occur through an increase in parenchymal and mammary fat pad weight, and parenchymal DNA content (an indicator of cell number).[24] Geiger and colleagues[25] also reported greater mammary epithelial cell (MEC) proliferation after weaning among calves fed a greater energy milk replacer before weaning, although others have found no effect of nutrition on mammary cell proliferation.[26,27] Postweaning, prepubertal mammary development is also affected by diet and impacts milk production in the subsequent lactation, although in an opposite direction to the effects of preweaning nutrition.[28] For example, dietary manipulation to enhance prepubertal weight gain in dairy heifers impairs mammogenesis and decreases subsequent milk yield,[29] which is at least partially attributed to changes in mammogenic hormone secretion.[30] In addition, greater average daily gains result in heifers attaining puberty at a younger age, which truncates the allometric growth phase of mammogenesis.[27] Together these studies suggest mammary ductal and fat pad development, before the first pregnancy, are critical for secretory tissue development during pregnancy and mammary function postpartum.[31–33] But, how these developmental processes might be influenced by environmental factors such as heat stress remains unknown.

HEAT STRESS AND MAMMARY DEVELOPMENT AND FUNCTION

Factors experienced early in life, such as disease, nutrition, and management interventions, can influence the lactation performance of heifers.[34] Of particular concern is environmental heat stress. Adverse effects of high temperatures on mammary development and function have been demonstrated both in vitro and in vivo. Bovine MEC growth, as estimated by DNA content, branching morphogenesis, and ductal branch extension is completely halted over a 24-hour period of exposure to high temperature in vitro.[35] Subjecting bovine MEC to a high incubation temperature for just 1 hour induces changes in cell ultrastructure characteristic of apoptosis, including chromatin condensation, formation of apoptotic bodies, and the presence of secondary lysosomes.[36] Moreover, increases in the proportion of MEC undergoing apoptosis and necrosis and decreases in cell viability and proliferation are detected after acute heat stress of both bovine and buffalo MEC in vitro.[36–38] In dairy cattle in vivo, dry pregnant cows exposed to heat stress have lower mammary cell proliferation relative to cows provided with active cooling.[11] The capacity of the lactating mammary gland to synthesize milk is a product of the number and metabolic activity of the secretory epithelial cells.[39] Thus, the inhibition of proliferation and increased cell death via apoptosis and necrosis likely contribute to reduced milk yield among heat-stressed cows.

Changes in molecular events in response to heat exposure have also been reported. Bovine MEC incubated briefly at high temperature upregulate expression of genes in the heat shock protein family.[35,37] Collier and colleagues[35] found that heat shock protein-70 gene expression increases up to approximately 4 hours after heat stress initiation followed by a sharp decrease to basal expression level concurrent with an increase in expression of proapoptotic genes. This decreases suggests thermotolerance loss as the duration of heat exposure increases. Similarly, the exposure of cultured buffalo MEC to high temperature induces changes in the expression of genes involved in apoptosis.[38] *BAX*, a proapoptotic gene, was upregulated, whereas, *BCL-2*, an antiapoptotic gene, and *IGFBP-5* were downregulated. IGFBP-5 is involved in tissue turnover by reducing the availability of IGF-1 and by its involvement in apoptosis via promotion of extracellular matrix degradation.[40] Also, IGFBP-5 increases in response to prolactin, which is higher in systemic circulation of heat-stressed, dry cows in vivo.[10,41] Shortly after heat stress initiation, bovine MEC increase expression of genes and proteins involved in the stress response and DNA and protein repair, with a downregulation of genes associated with the cell cycle, differentiation, the cytoskeleton, and milk synthesis.[35,37] Likewise, bovine MEC exposed to acute thermal stress have a lower expression of fatty acid synthase and several casein proteins, as well as lower concentrations of fatty acid synthase and beta casein in the culture media, indicative of milk synthesis impediment.[42] However, these results were not replicated in an in vivo study of heat-stressed dry cows, which did not detect differences in the expression of several genes involved in milk synthesis.[14] These empirical studies have contributed to our understanding of the cellular and molecular events occurring in mammary tissue after heat stress exposure.

Our recent transcriptomics analysis of mammary glands harvested from heat stressed or cooled dry cows, further support an effect of heat stress on mammary gland development and function.[43] Enrichment analysis of differentially expressed genes revealed that genes impacted by heat stress play a role in key processes in mammary gland development and health, such as ductal branching morphogenesis, extracellular matrix remodeling, cell death and proliferation, immune function, inflammation, and protection from cellular stress. The involvement of epithelial cell cilia in ductal branching morphogenesis is mediated by signaling pathways, such as Wnt and Sonic Hedgehog. Several genes in these pathways, including WIF1, LCA5, and MYO3B, were downregulated in the mammary gland of heat-stressed cows during the initial 14 days of the dry period. Moreover, we found upstream regulators and target genes involved in branching morphogenesis were negatively impacted by heat stress. This study is the first to directly link these genes and physiologic functions to an in vivo heat-stressed bovine model. Several genes associated with extracellular matrix degradation, such as MMP7 and MMP16, apoptosis, and lysosomal activity were downregulated, whereas Hsp40 was upregulated. The latter is congruent with reports of enhanced expression of genes and proteins in the heat shock family in bovine MEC in vitro when exposed to a thermal insult.

IN UTERO HEAT STRESS EFFECTS ON MAMMARY DEVELOPMENT AND FUNCTION

Heat stress also exerts transgenerational effects on the subsequent generation of heifers born to cows that experience heat stress in late gestation. The fetus can be affected by maternal heat stress through the intrauterine environment. Across 5 years of studies by our group, heifers born to dams that were heat stressed during late gestation were smaller through 1 year of age and produced significantly less milk (ie, 5 kg/d) in their first lactation relative to heifers born to dams that were cooled during late gestation, despite their similar age and weight at calving.[44] A more recent metaanalysis of 9 years of heat stress studies using the same experimental design (late gestation cows that experienced cooling or heat stress) confirmed that heat-stressed late gestation cows produce less milk during the subsequent lactation (**Fig. 1**A) and revealed in utero heat-stressed heifers produce significantly less milk during their first and second lactations, approximately 3.5 kg/d less, relative to in utero cooled heifers (**Fig. 1**B, C).[45] Through a preliminary study, we found in utero heat-stressed heifers have smaller mammary alveoli composed of fewer milk-producing cells during their first lactation relative to heifers born to cooled dams, which likely contributes to their poorer lactation performance.[46] Results of these studies point to effects of in utero heat stress on early mammary development that impair future growth, structure, and function.

To assess whether the thermal conditions experienced as a fetus alters tissue structure and cellular processes in the mammary gland, we harvested mammary biopsies from heifers (eg, gestated by heat stressed or cooled dams) at 21 and 42 days into their first lactation (entailing the early rising phase of milk yield and peak lactation, respectively).[46] Using immunohistochemistry techniques, we estimated the proportion

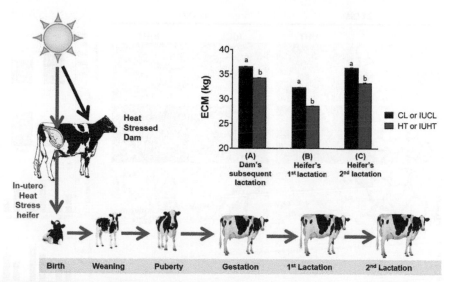

Fig. 1. (*A*) Dam energy-corrected milk yield (ECM) during subsequent lactation if under heat stress (HT, shade only; *orange bars*) or cooling (CL, fans and soakers; *blue bars*) when dry (approximately 46 days before calving). (*B*) First and (*C*) second lactation ECM of heifers born to heat stressed (IUHT, *orange bars*) or cooled dams (IUCL, *blue bars*). Different letters indicate significant differences between groups (*P*<.05).

of cells undergoing apoptosis and proliferation, the 2 main cell processes responsible for cell turnover in the lactating mammary gland.[47] The mammary glands of in utero heat-stressed heifers had alveoli with smaller luminal area compared with in utero cooled heifers, although the mammary alveoli number was similar between groups (**Fig. 2**). In addition, mammary glands of in utero heat-stressed heifers tended to contain a higher proportion of stromal connective tissue.

Alveolar size was associated with the number of secretory cells; smaller alveoli had fewer secretory epithelial cells. Thus, the mammary glands of in utero heat-stressed heifers had lower milk secretory capacity. In utero heat-stressed heifers had a lower percent of proliferating mammary cells, but no effect on the number of cells undergoing apoptosis (see **Fig. 2**).[46] Similarly, Tao and colleagues[11] documented reduced cell proliferation among heat-stressed, late gestation cows. Importantly, the disparity in mammary tissue morphology between in utero heat-stressed and in utero cooled heifers was not attributed to differences in the time available for secretory tissue growth and differentiation during gestation because both in utero heat-stressed and in utero cooled heifers had average gestation durations of 237 days. Likewise, differences in mammary structure were not attributed to disparities in thermal load during lactation or calf birth weight, because rectal temperatures, respiration rates, and calf birth weights were similar between in utero heat-stressed and cooled heifers. Overall, these studies suggest that an unfavorable intrauterine environment initiates aberrant mammary development that persists at least through the second lactation, more than 2 years after the insult.

Influences of the early life environment on offspring phenotype are often mediated by epigenetic modifications, such as DNA methylation, that regulate tissue-specific gene expression. In the mammary gland, the epigenome plays a critical role in the progressive commitment of mammary stem cells to specific progenitors and

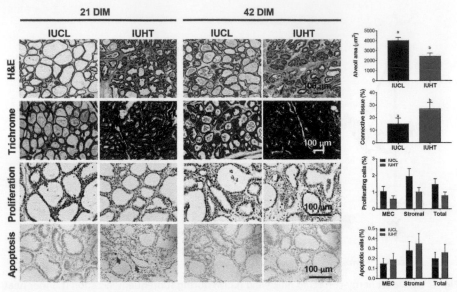

Fig. 2. Histology of mammary glands from first lactation heifers (21 and 42 days in milk [DIM]) born to heat stressed or cooled dams (IUHT vs IUCL). Mammary gland alveoli and connective tissue area (stain: hematoxylin and eosin and Masson's trichrome, respectively), percent of cells proliferating (Ki-67 assay), and percent of apoptotic cells (TUNEL assay). IUHT, *orange bars*; IUCL, *blue bars*. *Red arrows* indicate cells proliferating or undergoing apoptosis. Different letters indicate significant differences between groups (*P*<.05). (*From* Skibiel AL, Dado-Senn BM, Fabris TF, et al. In utero exposure to thermal stress has long-term effects on mammary gland microstructure and function in dairy cattle. PLoS One 2018b;13:e0206046, with permission.)

differentiated cells.[48] In addition, mammary cell maintenance and milk synthesis can be mediated by epigenetic mechanisms.[49] The growth and development of the liver, a key organ supporting the metabolic demands of copious milk secretion, is also modulated by the epigenome.[50] For these reasons, we examined the methylation profiles of mammary tissue harvested from in utero heat-stressed and cooled heifers during their first lactation and the liver of in utero heat-stressed and cooled bull calves at birth.[51] We identified more than 300 genes differentially methylated between the in utero heat-stressed and cooled groups associated with functions such as cell signaling, transcription, enzyme activation, immune function, cell proliferation, apoptosis, and development (**Fig. 3**). Heat stress induced changes in the epigenetic profiles of genes involved in proliferation, apoptosis, and development are particularly interesting in light of our histologic results (see **Fig. 2**) and our observation that many organs, including the liver, are lighter at birth in calves born to heat-stressed dams.[52,53] Notably, 50 of the differentially methylated genes identified were common to both heifer mammary gland and bull calf liver, suggesting that in utero heat stress may epigenetically program organs critical to lactation in a similar manner.

OTHER PHYSIOLOGIC IMPACTS OF IN UTERO HEAT STRESS

One of the clearest phenotypic observations made regarding in utero heat stress is a decrease in early life immune status; specifically, heat-stressed calves have lower circulating immunoglobulin concentrations compared with calves from cooled

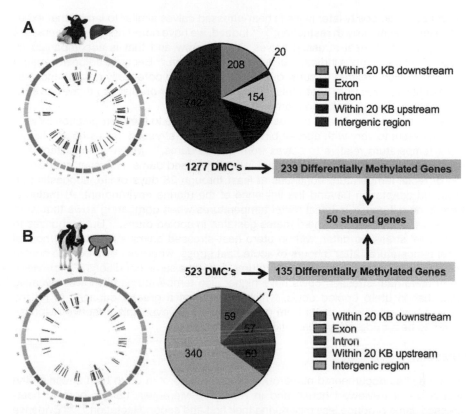

Fig. 3. Genomic and chromosomal locations of differentially methylated cytosines (DMCs) and genes (DMGs). Liver tissue was collected from in utero heat stressed and in utero cooled bull calves at birth. Mammary tissue was collected from in utero heat stressed and in utero cooled heifers at 21 days into their first lactation. Chromosomal and genomic location of DMGs and DMCs (*circular plot*) and genomic locations of DMCs (*pie graph*) for (*A*) bull calf liver and (*B*) heifer mammary gland.

dams.[54] We have shown that this response is not due to altered colostrum quality or IgG content, but rather is related to specific calf factors.[55] Further investigation supports the concept that in utero heat stress accelerates gut closure, thereby decreasing the capacity for IgG uptake regardless of the colostrum source.[53] Reduced IgG uptake owing to accelerated gut closure leads to lower immune status early in life, which is associated with poorer survival and a decreased number of heifers completing the first lactation after in utero heat stress.[44]

In utero heat stress alters endocrine systems with effects evident at birth and through early life that are consistent with metabolic adaptations to accumulate energy in peripheral tissues and reduce lean growth. Specifically, calves born to heat-stressed dams have greater circulating insulin in the first week of life relative to those born to cooled dams.[2] As calves that experience in utero heat stress develop, altered glucoregulatory responses are evident as illustrated by increased glucose clearance rate after a glucose tolerance test and insulin challenge relative to calves that were born to cooled dams. Of interest, circulating concentrations of cortisol at birth are increased in calves born to cooled dams relative to those from heat-stressed dams, but this effect dissipates quickly in early life.[54] Metabolic shifts may account for differences in adiposity later in life in heat-stressed calves similar to lambs that experience intrauterine growth restriction.[56,57] Indeed, we have noted persistent decreases in body weight in heat-stressed calves as they grow and that is accompanied by reduced stature, a gross indicator of lean mass accretion.[55] Because adiposity around puberty has been related to subsequent milk yield,[58] the potentially greater accumulation of fat in calves from heat-stressed dams may further predispose those calves to reduced milk yield and altered mammary growth.

Heat stress in utero clearly causes adaptive responses to thermoregulation as well, but they seem to vary with age. At birth, in utero heat-stressed calves have a higher rectal temperature relative to calves from cooled dams,[59] which is consistent with the elevated uterine temperature found in heat-stressed dams. However, that elevation of rectal temperature continues at least through 28 days of life, suggesting an extended adaptation beyond the influence of the uterine environment. At maturity, there is no difference in basal rectal temperatures when comparing cows that were heat stressed in utero with herd mates gestated in cooled dams.[52] But responses to acute heat stress do differ, with in utero heat-stressed animals maintaining normal rectal temperatures after 8 hours of acute heat stress, whereas cows born to cooled dams show increases in rectal temperatures under the same conditions. Functionally, the in utero heat-stressed cows have higher skin temperatures but lower sweating rates than in utero cooled cows, which may reflect a greater capacity to rid the body of heat relative to cows from cooled dams. However, this adaptive response seems to be a trade-off with lactation performance.

SUMMARY

Our group has documented numerous adverse effects of in utero heat stress on the postnatal calf (reviewed herein and in Refs.[2,60]). Moreover, heifers born to heat-stressed dams produce less milk during their first and second lactation.[44,45] Evidence from the literature and our preliminary data suggest in utero heat stress derails normal mammary development, which affects mammary growth throughout postnatal life, and ultimately impairs function. These shifts in mammary function are mirrored by altered endocrine, growth, and thermoregulatory responses. Accumulating evidence supports the concept that in utero heat stress programs a phenotype of reduced productivity at maturity in the dairy cow, and epigenetic mechanisms contribute to these morphologic and physiologic adaptations.

REFERENCES

1. Collier RJ, Dahl GE, VanBaale MJ. Major advances associated with environmental effects on dairy cattle. J Dairy Sci 2006;89:1244–53.
2. Tao S, Dahl GE. Heat stress effects during late gestation on dry cows and their calves. J Dairy Sci 2013;96:4079–93.
3. Bernabucci U, Lacetera N, Baumgard LH, et al. Metabolic and hormonal acclimation to heat stress in domesticated ruminants. Animal 2010;4:1167–83.
4. Hansen PJ. Genetic control of heat stress. Proc 49th Florida Dairy Prod Conf. Gainesville, Florida, March 16, 2013. p. 26–32.
5. Rhoads ML, Rhoads RP, VanBaale MJ, et al. Effects of heat stress and plane of nutrition on lactating Holstein cows: production, metabolism, and aspects of circulating somatotropin. J Dairy Sci 2009;92:1986–97.
6. Wheelock JB, Rhoads RP, VanBaale MJ, et al. Effects of heat stress on energetic metabolism in lactating Holstein cows. J Dairy Sci 2010;93:644–55.

7. St-Pierre NR, Cobanov B, Schnitkey G. Economic losses from heat stress by U.S. livestock industries. J Dairy Sci 2003;86(Suppl):E52–77.

8. Flamenbaum I. The beneficial effects of cooling cows. In: Proc. Cow Longevity Conf. Tumba, Sweden, August 28-29, 2013. p. 113–25.

9. Ferriera FC, Gennari RS, Dahl GE, et al. Economic feasibility of cooling dry cows across the United States. J Dairy Sci 2016;99:9931–41.

10. do Amaral BC, Connor EE, Tao S, et al. Heat-stress abatement during the dry period: does cooling improve transition into lactation? J Dairy Sci 2009;92: 5988–99.

11. Tao S, Bubolz JW, do Amaral BC, et al. Effect of heat stress during the dry period on mammary gland development. J Dairy Sci 2011;94:5976–86.

12. Tao S, Thompson IM, Monteiro APA, et al. Effect of cooling heat-stressed dairy cows during the dry period on insulin response. J Dairy Sci 2012;95:5035–46.

13. do Amaral BC, Connor EE, Tao S, et al. Heat stress abatement during the dry period influences metabolic gene expression and improves immune status in the transition period of dairy cows. J Dairy Sci 2011;94:86–96.

14. Tao S, Connor EE, Bubolz JW, et al. Effect of heat stress during the dry period on gene expression in mammary tissue and peripheral blood mononuclear cells. J Dairy Sci 2013;96:378–83.

15. Mejia C, Skibiel AL, Dado-Senn B, et al. Exposure of dairy cows to heat stress during late gestation or while in utero affects mammary gland microstructure. J Dairy Sci 2017;100(Suppl. 2):167 (Abstr.).

16. Skibiel AL, Zachut M, do Amaral BC, et al. Liver proteomic analysis of postpartum Holstein cows exposed to heat stress or cooling conditions during the dry period. J Dairy Sci 2018;101:705–16.

17. Wohlgemuth SE, Ramirez-Lee Y, Tao S, et al. Short Communication: effect of heat stress on mammary gland autophagy during the dry period. J Dairy Sci 2016;99: 4875–80.

18. Barker BJP, Eriksson JG, Forsén T, et al. Fetal origins of adult disease: strength of effects and biological basis. Int J Epidemiol 2002;31:1235–9.

19. McMillen IC, Robinson JS. Developmental origins of the metabolic syndrome: prediction, plasticity, and programming. Physiol Rev 2005;85:571–633.

20. Lucas A. Programming by early nutrition in man. Ciba Found Symp 1991;156: 38–55.

21. Mao WH, Albrecht E, Teuscher F, et al. Growth- and breed-related changes of fetal development in cattle. Asian-Australas J Anim Sci 2008;21:640–7.

22. van der Linden DS, Kenyon PR, Blair HT, et al. Effects of ewe size and nutrition on fetal mammary gland development and lactation performance. J Anim Sci 2009; 87:3944–54.

23. Soberon F, Raffrenato E, Everett RW, et al. Preweaning milk replacer intake and effects on long-term productivity of dairy calves. J Dairy Sci 2012;95:783–93.

24. Geiger AJ, Parsons CLM, Akers RM. Feeding a higher plane of nutrition and providing exogenous estrogen increases mammary gland development in Holstein heifer calves. J Dairy Sci 2016;99:7642–53.

25. Geiger AJ, Parsons CLM, Akers RM. Feeding an enhanced diet to Holstein heifers during the preweaning period alters steroid receptor expression and increases cellular proliferation. J Dairy Sci 2017;100:8534–43.

26. Brown EG, VandeHaar MJ, Daniels KM, et al. Effect of increasing energy and protein intake on mammary development in heifer calves. J Dairy Sci 2005;88: 595–603.

27. Meyer MJ, Capuco AV, Ross DA, et al. Developmental and nutritional regulation of the prepubertal bovine mammary gland: II. epithelial cell proliferation, parenchymal accretion rate, and allometric growth. J Dairy Sci 2006;89:4298–304.
28. Akers RM, McFadden TB, Purup S, et al. Local IGF-I axis in peripubertal ruminant mammary development. J Mammary Gland Biol Neoplasia 2000;5:43–51.
29. Sejrsen K, Purup S. Influence of prepubertal feeding level on milk yield potential of dairy heifers: a review. J Anim Sci 1997;75:828–35.
30. Sejrsen K, Huber JT, Tucker HA. Influence of amount fed on hormone concentrations and their relationship to mammary growth in heifers. J Dairy Sci 1983;66: 845–55.
31. Knight CH, Sorenson A. Windows in early mammary development: critical or not? Reproduction 2001;122:337–45.
32. Capuco AV, Ellis S, Wood DL, et al. Postnatal mammary ductal growth: three-dimensional imaging of cell proliferation, effects of estrogen treatment, and expression of steroid receptors in prepubertal calves. Tissue Cell 2002;34: 143–54.
33. Akers RM. Plasticity of mammary development in the prepubertal bovine mammary gland. J Anim Sci 2017;95:5653–63.
34. Heinrichs AJ, Heinrichs BS. A prospective study of calf factors affecting first-lactation and lifetime milk production and age of cows when removed from the herd. J Dairy Sci 2011;94:336–41.
35. Collier RJ, Stiening CM, Pollard BC, et al. Use of gene expression microarrays for evaluating environmental stress tolerance at the cellular level in cattle. J Anim Sci 2006;84(Suppl.):E1–13.
36. Du J, Di H-S, Guo L, et al. Hyperthermia causes bovine mammary epithelial cell death by a mitochondrial-induced pathway. J Therm Biol 2008;33:37–47.
37. Li L, Sun Y, Li X, et al. The global effect of heat on gene expression in cultured bovine mammary epithelial cells. Cell Stress Chaperones 2015;20:381–9.
38. Kapila N, Sharma A, Kishore A, et al. Impact of heat stress on cellular and transcriptional adaptation of mammary epithelial cells in riverine buffalo (Bubalus bubalis). PLoS One 2016;11:e0157237.
39. Capuco AV, Wood DL, Baldwin R, et al. Mammary cell number, proliferation, and apoptosis during a bovine lactation: relation to milk production and effect of bST. J Dairy Sci 2001;84:2177–87.
40. Nørgaard JV, Theil PK, Sørensen MT, et al. Cellular mechanisms in regulating mammary cell turnover during lactation and dry period in dairy cows. J Dairy Sci 2008;91:2319–27.
41. Collier RJ, Beede DK, Thatcher WW, et al. Influences of environment and its modification on dairy animal health and production. J Dairy Sci 1982;65:2213–27.
42. Li L, Wang Y, Li C, et al. Proteomic analysis to unravel the effect of heat stress on gene expression and milk synthesis in bovine mammary epithelial cells. Anim Sci J 2017;88:2090–9.
43. Dado-Senn BM, Skibiel AL, Fabris TF, et al. RNA-Seq reveals novel genes and pathways involved in bovine mammary involution during the dry period and under environmental heat stress. Sci Rep 2018;8:11096.
44. Monteiro APA, Tao S, Thompson IMT, et al. In utero heat stress decreases calf survival and performance through the first lactation. J Dairy Sci 2016;99:8443–50.
45. Laporta J, Ferreira FC, Dado-Senn B, et al. Dry period heat stress reduces dam, daughter, and granddaughter productivity. J Dairy Sci 2018;101(Suppl. 2):151 (Abstr.).

46. Skibiel AL, Dado-Senn BM, Fabris TF, et al. In utero exposure to thermal stress has long-term effects on mammary gland microstructure and function in dairy cattle. PLoS One 2018;13:e0206046.
47. Knight CH. The importance of cell division in udder development and lactation. Livest Prod Sci 2000;66:169–76.
48. Visvader JE, Stingl J. Mammary stem cells and the differentiation hierarchy: current status and perspectives. Genes Dev 2014;28:1143–58.
49. Singh K, Molenaar AJ, Swanson KM, et al. Epigenetics: a possible role in acute and transgenerational regulation of dairy cow milk production. Animal 2012;6: 375–81.
50. Snykers S, Henkens T, De Rop E, et al. Role of epigenetics in liver-specific gene transcription, hepatocyte differentiation and stem cell reprogrammation. J Hepatol 2009;51:187–211.
51. Skibiel AL, Peñagaricano F, Rocio A, et al. In utero heat stress alters the offspring epigenome. Sci Rep 2018;8:14609.
52. Ahmed BMS, Younas U, Asar TO, et al. Cows exposed to heat stress during fetal life exhibit improved thermal tolerance. J Anim Sci 2017;95:3497–503.
53. Ahmed BMS, Younas U, Asar TO, et al. Maternal heat stress reduces body and organ growth in calves: relationship to immune tissue development. J Dairy Sci 2016;99:606 (Abstr.).
54. Tao S, Monteiro AP, Thompson IM, et al. Effect of late-gestation maternal heat stress on growth and immune function of dairy calves. J Dairy Sci 2012;95: 7128–36.
55. Monteiro APA, Tao S, Thompson IMT, et al. Effect of heat stress during late gestation on immune function and growth performance of calves: isolation of altered colostral and calf factors. J Dairy Sci 2014;97:6426–39.
56. Morrison JL. Sheep models of intrauterine growth restriction: fetal adaptations and consequences. Clin Exp Pharmacol Physiol 2008;35:730–43.
57. Yates DT, Green AS, Limesand SW. Catecholamines mediate multiple fetal adaptations during placental insufficiency that contribute to intrauterine growth restriction: lessons from hyperthermic sheep. J Pregnancy 2011;2011:740408.
58. Silva LF, VandeHaar MJ, Whitlock BK, et al. Short communication: relationship between body growth and mammary development in dairy heifers. J Dairy Sci 2002; 85:2600–2.
59. Laporta J, Fabris TF, Skibiel AL, et al. In-utero exposure to heat stress during late-gestation has prolonged effects on activity patterns and growth of dairy calves. J Dairy Sci 2017;100:2976–84.
60. Dahl GE, Tao S, Laporta J. Late gestation heat stress of dairy cattle programs dam and daughter milk production. J Anim Sci 2017;95:5701–10.

Multigenerational Effects

Andrew J. Roberts, PhD*, El Hamidi Hay, PhD

KEYWORDS

- Epigenetics • Nutrition • Growth • Reproduction
- Genetic by environment interaction

KEY POINTS

- A large body of data is accumulating that provides evidence of epigenetic mediation of environmental influences on physiologic traits in humans and other species.
- Epigenetic mediation of gene expression may be transferred (inherited) across generations.
- Potential exists for using epigenetic approaches on a population or herd-wide basis to improve production efficiency in limited nutritional environments.
- Epigenetic mediation of gene expression can alter estimates of genetic sources of variation (genetic by environment interactions).

INTRODUCTION

The idea that environmental alterations of a phenotype are transferred across generations has existed for centuries.[1] In 1809, Lamarck postulated environmentally induced changes in a phenotype were passed on to subsequent generations. In 1859, Darwin proposed the concept of natural selection, in which the best-fit phenotype for a specific environment maintained a reproductive or survival advantage in that environment. Debates about whether inheritance of acquired characteristics or survival of the fittest was correct ensued throughout the nineteenth century. Weismann's experiment in the late 1800s showing that amputation of mice tails over 20 generations failed to alter tail length was considered strong evidence against the inheritance of acquired characteristics theory. In addition, the rediscovery of Mendel's work in the early 1900s provided insight into the mechanisms of inheritance and focused subsequent research toward understanding the genetic control of a phenotype. This resulted in the discovery of DNA and its role as the blueprint for life. Ultimately, genome sequencing ensued as the final step in understanding phenotypic diversity. However,

Disclosure statement: This work was funded by USDA appropriated funds (CRIS # 3030-31000-018-00D).
USDA, ARS, Fort Keogh Livestock and Range Research Laboratory, 243 Fort Keogh Road, Miles City, MT 59301, USA
* Corresponding author.
E-mail address: Andy.roberts@ars.usda.gov

the high levels of DNA sequence homology, within and across species, and lower than expected numbers of genes identified for numerous species has raised questions about whether DNA sequence variation is sufficient to explain the existing phenotypic variation or if other mechanisms may be contributing.

Data accumulated over the last 20 years support the concept that epigenetics mediates environmentally induced changes in a phenotype across generations. Epigenetic modification of the genome over and above alterations in nucleotide sequence is now considered a major factor contributing to different patterns of gene expression in different cell groups.[2] Inheritance of epigenetic modifications of gene expression across generations provides for phenotypic plasticity in the face of fixed genotype. Better understanding of epigenetic actions has resulted in a unified theory of evolution. This theory considers genotypic and epigenetic pathways for mediating environmental changes in a phenotype.[3] Although most epigenetics research has focused on the detrimental effects of nutritional deficiencies or environmental toxins, the natural role for epigenetics is adaptation to environment. Greater understanding and characterization of epigenetic responses to various management practices can enhance livestock production efficiency. This article briefly summarizes research on generational inheritance and provides examples of how this process may enhance the efficiency of beef cattle production.

Epigenetics Mediates Multigenerational Impacts of Environment

"Intergenerational factors may be defined as those factors, conditions, exposures, and environments experienced by one generation that relate to the health, growth, and development of the next generation."[4] Environmental factors may alter a phenotype via direct effect on the animal (first generation), direct or maternally mediated effects on the fetus (second generation), or gonadal cell lines of the fetus (third generation) when pregnant animals are exposed to environmental factors (fetal programming), and through inheritance across generations.[2,5] Epigenetic mediation of gene expression is a process contributing to the transfer of environmental impacts across generations.

In fetal programming, in which exposure of pregnant females to environmental stimuli influences the phenotypic traits observed in the fetus and the subsequent generation, the epigenetic change observed may be due to a direct or maternally mediated effect on the fetus and germ cells within the fetus, and not due to cross-generational inheritance.[5] In addition, the physiologic processes influenced by fetal programming depend on when exposure to environmental stimuli occurs with respect to conception or stage of embryonic or fetal development, and embryonic or fetal sex.[3,6,7]

Obviously, the generational interval of a species markedly influences the capacity to study the mutigenerational impacts of environmental factors. Much of the research evaluating multigenerational effects has focused on nutritional deficiencies, diseases, and other undesirable responses. Research demonstrating generational impacts on human offspring from populations subjected to extreme nutritional stress led to the thrifty phenotype hypothesis.[8] This hypothesis proposes that mothers subjected to nutritional deficiencies forecast the environment their offspring will be born in, thereby providing their offspring with a survival advantage. Exposure of females to severe nutritional deficiency during pregnancy results in altered metabolism and provides enhanced capacity for caloric storage in offspring later in life. This hypothesis has led to many studies using laboratory and domestic animals as models to facilitate tight control of dietary treatments at specific stages of pregnancy. These studies provide insight into the physiologic mechanisms that mediate the impact of undernutrition and overnutrition during fetal development at specific time points later in life.[9–11] Although the thrifty phenotype hypothesis implied survival advantage in nutritionally limited environments, the metabolic changes identified in these studies resulted in undesirable health consequences in offspring existing in ample nutrient environments.[8] For example, indigenous populations that evolved under seasonal periods of feast and famine exhibit high instances of metabolic disorder after changing to a more sedentary lifestyle.[2]

Although it is logical that the thrifty phenotype hypothesis would apply to wild animal populations,[12] the extent that it may apply to the more highly managed livestock industry has not been thoroughly evaluated. Animals within a herd are all subjected to similar environmental stimuli throughout the production cycle; any stimuli resulting in epigenetic modification may result in herd-wide changes. The cumulative effects of herd-wide exposure and generational inheritance are rapid changes in phenotypic characteristics of the population when compared with the rate of phenotypic change brought about by genetic selection.

Relative to the poultry, swine, and dairy industries, beef and lamb production occurs with less management of the production environment. Therefore, species managed under pastoral grazing systems may be more influenced by epigenetic alterations of gene expression. At present, the impact of epigenetics in any of the livestock industries has not been well-described. However, increased awareness of the potential generational effects associated with epigenetics has led to greater consideration about how relatively small nutritional differences imposed under common production practices may lead to metabolic programming that alters the production characteristics of the offspring.[7,13] Due to long generation intervals, much of this research has been limited to evaluating the impacts of uterine programming on the postnatal characteristics of the gestating fetus or the direct effects of nutritional impacts during postnatal development. Studies following the multigenerational effects are scarce. The limited studies on cattle populations managed under extensive environments for long periods of time indicate a metabolic adaptive response, resulting in their ability to function below National Research Council (NRC)[14] requirements.[15] Collectively, the research indicates the potential to propagate desired characteristics in the livestock industry through epigenetic pathways.

An example of how long-term differences in nutritional management may result in differences in multigenerational responses to nutritional restriction is provided by Vonnahme and colleagues.[16] These researchers evaluated response to nutritional restriction in ewes originating from a common genetic population but managed for several generations under very different nutritional environments. Ewes maintained in a relatively sedentary lifestyle with a diet that always met or exceeded NRC recommendations exhibited greater loss in bodyweight and body condition score (BCS), and greater suppression in placental efficiency and fetal growth in response to nutritional restriction, than ewes from a herd maintained in an extensive, semiarid range environment. Thus, long-term differences in nutritional management resulted in a divergence in response to short-term nutritional restriction. Whether these differences are driven by divergence in selection or epigenetic modulation is not known. These results support the concept that management under divergent nutritional environments alters nutritional requirements and response to nutritional limitations in subsequent generations.

Example of Multigenerational Effects in Cattle from a Lifetime Productivity Study

In 2001, a long-term research project was initiated at the US Department of Agriculture, Agriculture Research Service, Fort Keogh Livestock and Range Research

Laboratory, Miles City, Montana, to study the lifelong impact of feeding 1 of 2 levels of protein supplementation to cows grazing dormant winter pasture during the last trimester of gestation. It was hypothesized that management with lesser inputs over time would provide selection pressure for more efficient cows. Two possible modes of action leading to support of the hypothesis would be (1) a change in genetic composition of the herd or (2) a metabolic adaptation to function with less input. Genetic change would require a long period of time compared with metabolic adaptation. The adaptation process could also result in altered uterine function, bringing about epigenetic changes in the offspring.

Detailed description of the study and the most recent summary of results are available from Roberts and colleagues[13] (2016). Following is a brief description of the treatments and some of the previously published results. In December of each winter, cows were divided into their lifelong assigned treatment group, which was predicted to provide a marginal (MARG) or adequate (ADEQ) level of protein supplementation based on NRC requirements. They were supplemented with either 1.1 kg/d (MARG, n = 138 cows and 21 bred heifers) or 1.8 kg/d (ADEQ, n = 92 cows and 19 bred heifers) of alfalfa hay. To remain in the population, cows were required to get pregnant and wean a calf each year. When analyzed over 9 years, differences in the supplemental feed levels resulted in the ADEQ-supplemented cows gaining more weight during supplementation than MARG-supplemented cows (least squares means for age-adjusted differences over 9 years were 25 ± 1.3 vs 22 ± 1.2 kg weight change for ADEQ vs MARG levels, P<.05). This difference was accompanied by differences in BCS at precalving between the ADEQ-supplemented cows (4.98 ± 0.04) and the MARG-supplemented cows (4.86 ± 0.03, BCS scale of 1 = extremely thin to 9 = extremely fat, P<.02). Pregnancy rates over the 2002 to 2007 breeding seasons were 92 plus or minus 1.9% and 91 plus or minus 1.6% for the ADEQ and MARG level groups, respectively (P = .8).[13] Thus, the difference in supplementation resulted in a small divergence in weight change over the last trimester of pregnancy but did not affect pregnancy rates. For subsequent discussion, animals from this portion of the study are referred to as the first generation.

Heifers born in the study from 2002 to 2011 were allotted by weaning weight within dam treatment to be fed to appetite (control, n = 656) or fed at 80% of that consumed by control heifers at a common bodyweight basis (restricted, n = 655) over a 140-day period between weaning and first breeding. Heifers were exposed for breeding and pregnant heifers were retained for replacement. As with the first generation, the replacement females grazed dormant winter forage each year. Control heifers were supplemented each winter with 1.8 kg/d protein supplement and restricted heifers were provided 1.1 kg/d treatments, corresponding to the ADEQ and MARG levels of supplement, respectively. These females represented daughters of the first generation, as well as subsequent generations. With 1 exception, previous analyses of the data have been limited to the classification by individual treatment and dam treatment (ie, 2 × 2 for most recent generations).[13] Thus, previously published results did not differentiate between second and third generation females (see later discussion). In previous analyses, the main effects of dam treatment during the last trimester of pregnancy were observed for bodyweights on daughters at 3 years of age and older. Females born to MARG-supplemented dams were heavier at the start of breeding at 3 years and older, and had greater BCS than females from the ADEQ-supplemented dams. The difference in weight at 3 years of age was associated with greater retention (less loss due to reproductive failure) between 3 and 4 years of age. Interaction of dam treatment and individual treatment were observed for the calves produced by the cows, the only third-generation trait previously analyzed. Restricted cows from

MARG-supplemented dams produced lighter calves at birth and weaning than their contemporary herd mates.

For statistical purposes, in the remaining portion of this article, the differentiation of second-generation and third-generation females is accomplished by treatment coding of the maternal granddam (MGD). Animals were considered second-generation females if their MGD was not subjected to the different supplementation levels, whereas any female whose MGD was subjected to either ADEQ or MARG winter supplementation was classified as a third-generation female. Note that this classification method for the third generation does not differentiate between females with treatments applied for more than 3 generations. This classification process allowed analysis of the generational effects of the 2 treatment levels applied to the last 3 generations (individual treatment, dam treatment, and MGD treatment). In addition, sires used on this population were produced by females in the study, providing an opportunity to evaluate the impact of the supplement level provided to the sire's dam on each of the sire's daughters (ie, the paternal granddam [PGD] effect).

As previously discussed, earlier analyses indicated that the MGD treatment by dam treatment interaction on offspring weight at birth and weaning, in which offspring from MARG-supplemented dams out of MARG-supplemented dams, produced calves slightly smaller at birth and weaning when compared with other dam treatment by MGD treatment classifications.[13] These interactions were also evident in the most recent analyses conducted for this article (**Table 1**, analyzed for males and females). The current analyses indicate these lighter weights at birth and weaning were associated with shorter hip height in daughters at 1 year of age (see **Table 1**). The supplement level provided to the MGDs influenced the loin muscle area of granddaughters at 1 year of age (measured by carcass ultrasound) and weight at prebreeding at approximately 14 months of age. Heifers descending from the MARG-supplemented MGDs had smaller loin muscle area and were 5 kg lighter than heifers from the ADEQ-supplemented MGDs (see **Table 1**). A trend was also observed for the effect of dam treatment on heifer offspring weight at 14 months of age, with heifers out of the MARG-supplemented dams weighing 4 kg less than heifers out of the ADEQ-supplemented dams. As expected, the prebreeding weight of heifers was altered by the feeding level (control vs restricted) during postweaning development. Restricted feeding resulted in lighter prebreeding weights than control feeding (restricted and control are designated as MARG and ADEQ, respectively, in **Table 1**, based on winter supplementation level). The prebreeding weight of cows 5 years of age and older was influenced by interactions of MGD and dam treatments, and MGD and individual treatments (see **Table 1**). In previous analyses that did not include the MGD effects, the main effect of dam treatment and individual treatments were observed.[13] Cows out of MARG-supplemented dams were heavier than cows out of the ADEQ-supplemented dams. Animals receiving the ADEQ supplement each winter were heavier than cows given the MARG supplement (ie, direct effect of supplement level). The current results indicate an increase in mature weight occurred with MARG supplementation to either the MGD or dam, and that MGD treatment is important when evaluating the direct effect of supplement levels on weight change. Animals supplemented at the same level as their MGD were heavier than animals that received the opposite of the supplement treatment that their MGD received.

The supplement level provided to the PGD influenced heifer (granddaughter) intramuscular fat at 1 year of age, in which heifers descending from MARG-supplemented PGDs had greater intramuscular fat than heifers from the ADEQ-supplemented PGDs (see **Table 1**). The prebreeding weight of cows 5 years and older was influenced by the interaction of PGD and individual treatments (see

Table 1 Effect of supplementation level provided to paternal granddam, maternal granddam, dam, or individual on growth and ultrasound carcass measurements						
MGD Treatment	MARG[a]		ADEQ[a]			
Dam treatment	MARG	ADEQ	MARG	ADEQ	SE	P
Birth weight[b], kg	33.8[d]	34.5	34.3	34.5	0.17	.08
Weaning weight[b], kg	201[d]	215	214	214	1	<.01
Hip height at 12 mo age, cm	116[d]	118	117	117	0.3	<.01
MGD treatment	MARG	ADEQ				
Loin muscle area at 12 mo age, cm²	52.9	54.2	—	—	0.3	.01
PGD treatment	MARG	ADEQ				
Intramuscular fat at 12 mo age, %	3.7	3.5	—	—	0.02	.03
Weight at 14 mo age, kg	MARG	ADEQ				
Effect of MGD treatment	301	306	—	—	2	.03
Effect of dam treatment	302	306	—	—	2	.10
Effect of Individual treatment	296	311	—	—	2	<.01
MGD treatment	MARG		ADEQ			
Dam treatment	MARG	ADEQ	MARG	ADEQ		
Mature weight[c], kg	517	512	518	500[d]	5	.09
MGD treatment	MARG		ADEQ			
Individual treatment	MARG	ADEQ	MARG	ADEQ		
Mature weight[c], kg	524	505[d]	502[d]	516	5	<.01
PGD treatment	MARG		ADEQ			
Individual treatment	MARG	ADEQ	MARG	ADEQ		
Mature weight[c], kg	506[d]	514[d,e]	520[e]	507[d]	5	<.01

[a] Animals were provided either 1.1 kg/d (MARG) or 1.8 kg/d (ADEQ) alfalfa hay as supplement while grazing dormant native range during the last trimester of pregnancy. Rows with 4 values depict means for interactions of treatments indicated in preceding two rows. Rows with 2 values depict means for main effect of treatment indicated in preceding row.
[b] Some of these data were analyzed and reported previously.[13]
[c] Weight of cows 5 years and older taken before start of breeding, approximately 3 mo after ending the winter supplement treatment.
[d] Means in same row without similar superscripts differ (P<.05).
[e] Means in same row without similar superscripts differ (P<.05).

Table 1). Weight rankings in the PGD by individual treatment interaction are opposite of ranking in the MGD by individual treatment interaction. Cows fed the same level of supplement as their PGD were lighter than cows fed the opposite supplement treatment of their PGD.

The expanded model applied in the current analyses indicates transgenerational effects and a parental path of inheritance (ie, MGD vs PGD) must be considered when evaluating direct treatment effects on individuals, as well as carryover effects from dam treatments. The magnitude of differences reported in **Table 1** reflects a 2% to 4% difference in weight. This magnitude of difference is much lower than differences reported for many studies evaluating severe nutrition deficiencies.[2] Exposure of 2 successive generations to MARG supplementation resulted in offspring exhibiting reduced weights at birth through at least 1 year of age; however, weights later in life were greater in offspring descending from cows subjected to 1 or 2 generations of MARG supplementation. Although not presented, the differences in BCS paralleled the differences in mature weights, in which heavier weights were associated with a greater BCS. So, differences in weight reflect differences in body composition and not necessarily a change in body size. These results would be consistent with metabolic changes that result in a caloric storage advantage (see previous discussion), which may provide a reproductive advantage in limited environments.

Pregnancy rates at 3 years of age were influenced by the interaction of the MGD treatments by dam treatments (**Table 2**), with the lowest pregnancy rates occurring in cows coming from the ADEQ-supplemented dams and the ADEQ-supplemented MGDs. The pregnancy rate at 5 years of age was influenced by MGD treatment by individual treatment interaction (see **Table 2**), with the lowest pregnancy rates occurring in the ADEQ-supplemented cows from the ADEQ-supplemented MGDs. Although these results reflect positively for MARG supplementation, pregnancy success at specific ages is not independent from pregnancy rates at earlier ages. Rebreeding rates of 2-year-old females was decreased by the direct effect of MARG supplementation.[13] This potentially influences the population structure progressing to the next age, whereby less fit females may be culled out earlier in life under a MARG level of supplementation but not until older ages when managed under ADEQ supplementation. Continued data collection will provide greater insight into the generational impact on longevity. However, it is interesting to speculate that generational inheritance of environmentally stimulated changes in gene expression may be contributing to the genetic by environment interaction recently reported for stayability (measure of longevity) in cattle.[17]

Consideration of Epigenetics in Genetic by Environmental Interactions

Several livestock traits are under the control of genetic and environmental factors and their interaction. In today's application of genetics in the livestock industry, genetic by environment interactions are not generally considered. However, with the continued accumulation of data concerning how epigenetics may mediate environmental effects on gene expression, accounting for such effects is needed. Genetic by environment interactions have been widely studied. However, few studies have explored the effects of nutritional environments on the genetics of the animals and their offspring. Studying the effects of the environment on the genetic merit of the animal quantitatively could be carried out through 2 approaches. The first is a multitrait model that treats each observation of a given trait in a certain environment as different and assumes genetic correlations.[18–21] The second approach is using a reaction norm model that requires a continuous environmental gradient. This approach allows the characterization of the trajectory of animal performance across the environment.[22–26]

Table 2
Interaction of supplement level provided to maternal granddam and dam, or maternal granddam and individual, on pregnancy rate

MGD treatment	MARG[a]		ADEQ[a]			P
Dam treatment	MARG	ADEQ	MARG	ADEQ	SE	MGD × dam
% Pregnant at 3 y age	84[b,c]	85[b]	88[b]	75[b,c]	4	.065
Individual treatment	MARG	ADEQ	MARG	ADEQ	SE	MGD × individual
% Pregnant at 5 y age	93[b]	99[b]	96[b,c]	89[b,c]	3	.03

[a] Animals were provided either 1.1 kg/d (MARG) or 1.8 kg/d (ADEQ) alfalfa hay as supplement while grazing dormant native range during the last trimester of pregnancy.
[b] Means in same row without similar superscripts differ (P<.05).
[c] Means in same row without similar superscripts differ (P<.1).

Exploring how nutrition affects the genetics of an animal and its offspring was conducted by Hay and Roberts[27] (2018) using these 2 approaches. Results indicated genetic estimates for postweaning average daily gain (ADG) were subject to the interaction of nutritional environment imposed on the dam during pregnancy (ie, genetic by environment interaction, where environment was classified as ADEQ or MARG treatments; see previous discussion). Results indicated that the genetic estimate for ADG differed depending on prenatal environment. The results also indicated a higher impact of genetic by nutritional environment interaction on phenotypes with lower heritability. Genetic breeding values of the offspring showed a change in magnitude across the ADEQ and MARG treatments and, in some cases, reranking. Furthermore, the indirect genetic response to selection differed between the environments and, in some cases, lower nutritional input environments resulted in a higher genetic response. Although not directly established, differences resulting from fetal programming may account for the observed results. Unpublished results from a study by Hay and Roberts showed a change of single nucleotide polymorphisms (SNPs) effects in the offspring across the dam's nutritional environments (ADEQ and MARG supplementation). The percentage of maternal genetic variance explained by each SNP for birth weight differed between the MARG and the ADEQ supplemented groups. This difference was greatest for a SNP located on 24Mb on chromosome 14. This chromosome has been reported to harbor many genes and quantitative trait loci, controlling growth and metabolism.

With the existence of genetic by environment interaction, it is sensible to have environment-specific breeding programs. However, in beef cattle, most genetic evaluations are based on phenotypic data from a limited range of environments and seldom on animals having offspring in very different environments. Genomics could help with this issue because SNP could be used to compute genomic breeding values in different environments, which, in turn, could be used for selection and mating decisions. However, this would require a large genomic reference dataset spanning various environments.

SUMMARY

Environmental influences resulting in epigenetic mediation of gene expression can affect multiple generations via a direct effect on the animal; direct or maternally mediated effects on the fetus, or gonadal cell lines of the fetus when pregnant animals are exposed; and through inheritance across generations. Although much of the research on multigenerational effects has focused on nutritional deficiencies, diseases, and other undesirable responses, tremendous potential exists to use epigenetics as a tool to improve production efficiency. Because animals within a herd are all subjected to similar environmental stimuli throughout the production cycle, any stimuli resulting in epigenetic modification may result in herd-wide changes. Beef production occurs with less management of the production environment than swine, poultry, and dairy. This indicates beef production may be influenced to a greater extent by epigenetic alterations of gene expression than industries incorporating greater environmental control. Production practices that result in herd-wide exposure to specific nutritional environments, resulting in generational inheritance of desirable characteristics, will be much more rapid than pursuing phenotypic change through genetic selection. At present, the impact epigenetics has had in the livestock industry is not well-described. However, significant potential exists to propagate desired characteristics in the livestock industry through epigenetic pathways and these pathways may alter estimates of genetic variance (ie, expected progeny differences), thereby resulting in genetic by environment interactions that will need to be taken into consideration when using traditional genetic selection.

REFERENCES

1. Rothwell RV. Understanding genetics. 2nd edition. New York: Oxford University Press; 1979. p. 2–9.
2. Drake AJ, Walker BR. The intergenerational effects of fetal programming: non-genomic mechanisms for the inheritance of low birth weight and cardiovascular risk. J Endocrinol 2004;180:1–16.
3. Skinner MK. Environmental epigenetics and a unified theory of the molecular aspects of evolution: a Neo-Lamarckian concept that facilitates Neo-Darwinian evolution. Genome Biol Evol 2015;7(5):1296–302.
4. Emanuel I. Maternal health during childhood and later reproductive performance. Ann N Y Acad Sci 1986;477:27–39.
5. Nilsson EE, Skinner MK. Environmentally induced epigenetic transgenerational inheritance of reproductive disease. Biol Reprod 2015;93(6):145. http://www.bioone.org/doi/full/10.1095/biolreprod.115.134817.
6. Rhind SM, McKelvey WAC, McMillen S, et al. Effect of restricted food intake, before and/or after mating, on the reproductive performance of Greyface Ewes. Anim Prod 1989;48:149–55. https://doi.org/10.1017/S0003356100003883.
7. Funston RN, Summers AF. Epigenetics: setting up lifetime production of beef cows by managing nutrition. Annu Rev Anim Biosci 2013;1:339–63.
8. Hales CN, Barker DJ. The thrifty phenotype hypothesis. Br Med Bull 2001;60: 5–20. https://doi.org/10.1093/bmb/60.1.5.
9. Wu G, Bazer FW, Wallace JM, et al. Board invited review. Intrauterine growth retardation: implications for the animal sciences. J Anim Sci 2006;84:2316–37. https://doi.org/16908634.
10. Reynolds LP, Borowicz PP, Caton JS, et al. Developmental programming: the concept, large animal models, and the key role of uteroplacental vascular development. J Anim Sci 2010;88(E. Suppl):E61–72. https://doi.org/10.2527/jas.2009-2359.
11. Ford SP, Long NM. Evidence for similar changes in offspring phenotype following either maternal undernutrition or overnutrition: potential impact on fetal epigenetic mechanisms. Reprod Fertil Dev 2012;24:105–11. http://refhub.elsevier.com/S0749-0720(13)00053-4/sref29.
12. Marshall HH, Vitikainen EIK, Mwanguhya F, et al. Lifetime fitness consequences of early-life ecological hardship in a wild mammal population. Ecol Evol 2017; 7(6):1712–24. https://doi.org/10.1002/ece3.2747.
13. Roberts AJ, Funston RN, Grings EE, et al. TRIENNIAL REPRODUCTION SYMPOSIUM: Beef Heifer development and lifetime productivity in rangeland-based production systems. J Anim Sci 2016;94:2705–15. https://doi.org/10.2527/jas.2016-0435.
14. NRC. Nutrient requirements of beef cattle. 7th 514 rev. edition. Washington, DC: Natl. Acad. Press; 2000. p. 515.
15. Petersen MK, Mueller CJ, Mulliniks JT, et al. BEEF SPECIES SYMPOSIUM: potential limitations of NRC in predicting energetic requirements of beef females within western U.S. grazing systems. J Anim Sci 2014;92:2800–8. https://doi.org/10.2527/jas.2013-7310.

16. Vonnahme KA, Hess BW, Nijland MJ, et al. Placentomal differentiation may compensate for maternal nutrient restriction in ewes adapted to harsh range conditions. J Anim Sci 2006;84:3451–9. https://doi.org/10.2527/jas.2006-132.

17. Fennewald DJ, Weaber RL, Lamberson WR. Genotype by environment interaction for stayability of Red Angus in the United States. J Anim Sci 2018;96:422–9.

18. Hayes BJ, Carrick M, Bowman P, et al. Genotype × environment interaction for milk production of daughters of Australian dairy sires from test-day records. J Dairy Sci 2003;86:3736–44. https://doi.org/10.3168/jds.S0022-0302(03)73980-0.

19. Mulder H, Bijma P. Effects of genotype × environment interaction on genetic gain in breeding programs. J Anim Sci 2005;83:49–61. https://doi.org/10.2527/2005.83149x.

20. Williams J, Bertrand J, Misztal I, et al. Genotype by environment interaction for growth due to altitude in United States Angus cattle. J Anim Sci 2012;90:2152–8. https://doi.org/10.2527/jas.2011-4365.

21. Raidan F, Passafaro TL, Fragomeni BO, et al. Genotype × environment interaction in individual performance and progeny tests in beef cattle. J Anim Sci 2015;93:920–33. https://doi.org/10.2527/jas.2014-7983.

22. Ravagnolo O, Misztal I. Genetic component of heat stress in dairy cattle, parameter estimation. J Dairy Sci 2000;83:2126–30. https://doi.org/10.3168/jds.S0022-0302(00)75095-8.

23. Pegolo NT, Albuquerque LG, Lôbo R, et al. Effects of sex and age on genotype × environment interaction for beef cattle body weight studied using reaction norm models. J Anim Sci 2011;89:3410–25. https://doi.org/10.2527/jas.2010-3520.

24. Cardoso F, Tempelman R. Linear reaction norm models for genetic merit prediction of Angus cattle under genotype by environment interaction. J Anim Sci 2012;90:2130–41. https://doi.org/10.2527/jas.2011-4333.

25. Hammami H, Vandenplas J, Vanrobays ML, et al. Genetic analysis of heat stress effects on yield traits, udder health, and fatty acids of Walloon Holstein cows. J Dairy Sci 2015;98:4956–68. https://doi.org/10.3168/jds.2014-9148.

26. Fennewald DJ, Weaber RL, Lamberson W. Genotype by environment interactions for growth in Red Angus. J Anim Sci 2017;95:538–44. https://doi.org/10.2527/jas.2016.0846.

27. Hay EH, Roberts A. Genotype × prenatal and post-weaning nutritional environment interaction in a composite beef cattle breed using reaction norms and multi-trait model. J Anim Sci 2018;96:444–53. https://doi.org/10.1093/jas/skx057.

Developmental Resiliency
In Utero Adaption to Environmental Stimuli

Adam F. Summers, PhD*, Eric J. Scholljegerdes, PhD

KEYWORDS

- Fetal programming • Maternal nutrition • Environmental adaptation • Livestock

KEY POINTS

- Prediction of intake in grazing-based systems can be challenging and may explain variation in results from fetal programming-based research.
- Maternal environmental conditions may program progeny for improved performance through various mechanisms.
- Severe nutrient restriction (<50% of requirements) seems to be necessary for consistent results in various studies.

INTRODUCTION

The use of nutritional programs to compensate for dietary limitations is a normal part of livestock production. Feeding accounts for a large portion of annual production costs, thus producers often seek ways to reduce inputs. Historically, producers would allow for cyclical body weight (BW) changes in dams. However, the understanding of fetal programming has put this practice into question. The understanding of fetal programming or developmental programming indicates that nutritional or environmental stressors during pregnancy can have lasting effects on subsequent progeny.[1–3] In most but not all cases, postnatal outcomes are poorer than well-fed contemporaries (**Table 1**). However, there are instances in which the nutrient-deprived treatment outperformed the seemingly well-fed group. What remains to be fully elucidated is the underlying mechanisms that cause a positive versus a negative outcome in developmental programming research. Likewise, can an animal be overfed to improve productivity and is there a particular nutrient that is more impactful?

Grazing

In an effort to model real-world environments, research must be conducted outside of the well-controlled feeding studies because almost all offspring are gestated by dams

The authors have nothing to disclose.
Department of Animal and Range Sciences, New Mexico State University, P. O. Box 30003, Las Cruces, NM 88003, USA
* Corresponding author.
E-mail addresses: asummers@nmsu.edu; ejs@nmsu.edu

Table 1
Effects of gestational nutrition on progeny performance

Reference	Feeding Period	Grazing or Dry Lot	Diet[a]	Treatment[b]	Progeny Response							
					Birth BW	WW	Prebreeding BW/YW/ Finish BW[c]	Carcass Quality[d]	Feed Efficiency[e]	Age at Puberty	Pregnancy %[f]	Calved in 1st 21 d
Bohnert et al,[39] 2013	Late gest	Fed 6% CP meadow hay on pasture	No DDGS vs DDGS	—	↓	↓	ND	ND	—	—	—	—
	—	—	—	BCS 4 vs BCS 6	↓	ND	ND	ND	—	—	—	—
Funston et al,[9] 2010	Late gest	Grazing	Corn residue vs winter range	—	ND	↑	ND	—	↓	ND	ND	ND
	—	—	No suppl vs 0.4 kg 31% CP	—	ND	↑	ND	—	↑	ND	ND	ND
Larson et al,[8] 2009	Late gest	Grazing	Corn residue vs winter range	—	↑	↑	ND	↑	ND	—	—	—
	—	—	No suppl vs 0.45 kg 28% CP	—	ND	↑	↑	↑	ND	—	—	—
Long et al,[40] 2010	Early gest: d 32–115	Dry lot for 55% Grazing for 100%	55% vs 100% NRC req	—	ND	ND	ND	ND	ND	ND	ND	—
Long et al,[41] 2010	60 d before pregnancy through parturition	Dry lot (ewes)	150% vs 100% NRC req	—	↑	—	—	—	ND	—	—	—
Long et al,[20] 2012	Early to late gest	Dry lot	70% vs 100% NRC req	—	—	—	ND	—	—	—	—	—

Study	Gestation	Management	Treatment	Comparison							
Marques et al,[42] 2016	Late gest	Dry lot	Mixture	—	ND	ND	ND	—	—	—	—
Marques et al,[22] 2016	Early to late gest	Mixture	—	Low vs high BCS	ND	—	—	—	—	—	—
				BCS gained 1st trimester vs high BCS	ND	—	—	—	—	—	—
				BCS gained 2nd trimester vs high BCS	↑	—	—	—	—	—	—
				BCS gained 3rd trimester vs high BCS	↑	—	—	—	—	—	—
Martin et al,[6] 2007	Late gest	Grazing	Protein vs No protein suppl	—	ND	↑	—	ND	ND	↑	↑
Micke et al,[23] 2010	Early and mid gest	Dry lot	240% vs 70% CP req in early gest	—	ND	↓♂ ↑♀	ND	—	—	—	—
			240% vs 70% CP req in mid gest	—	↑	ND	ND	—	—	—	—
Mohrhauser et al.[10] 2015	Mid gest	Grazing and dry lot	Grazing: 100% req Dry lot 80% req	—	—	—	ND	—	—	—	—
Mulliniks et al,[27] 2016	Late gest	Grazing	—	Loss of BCS vs moderate or high gain of BCS	ND	ND	↑	—	—	—	—
Shoup et al,[24] 2015	Late gest	Grazing	No suppl vs low or high CP suppl	Early vs normal wean time	ND	Early wean: low ↑ High: ND Normal: ND	—	ND	—	—	—
Shoup et al,[28] 2015	Late gest	Grazing	No suppl vs low or high CP suppl	Early vs normal wean time	—	ND	ND	—	—	—	—

(continued on next page)

Table 1
(continued)

Reference	Feeding Period	Grazing or Dry Lot	Diet[a]	Treatment[b]	Birth BW	WW	Prebreeding BW/YW/ Finish BW[c]	Carcass Quality[d]	Feed Efficiency[e]	Age at Puberty	Pregnancy %[f]	Calved in 1st 21 d
							Progeny Response					
Shoup et al,[43] 2016	Late gest	Grazing	Endophyte free vs infected	—	ND	ND	ND	ND	ND	—	—	—
Summers et al,[31,32] 2015	Late gest	Dry lot	No suppl vs high or low RUP	—	ND	ND	ND	ND	ND	—	—	—
Stalker et al,[5] 2006	Late gest	Grazing	CP suppl vs no suppl	—	ND	↑	—	ND	—	—	—	—
Taylor et al,[11] 2016	Mid gest	Grazing and dry lot	Grazing – 100% req vs Dry lot – 80% req	—	ND	ND	ND	—	ND	—	—	—
Wilson et al,[30] 2015	Late gest	Dry lot	Low RDP vs high RDP	—	↑	ND	ND	ND	ND	—	—	—
Wilson et al,[33] 2016	Mid to late gest	Dry lot	125% NRC TDN req vs 100%	—	↑	↑	ND	ND	ND	—	—	—
Wilson et al,[44] 2016	Late gest	Dry lot	129% NRC CP req vs 100%	—	ND	ND	ND	ND	ND	—	—	—

Abbreviations: BCS, body condition score; CP, crude protein; DDGS, dried distillers grains with solubles; gest, gestation; ND, not different; NRC, National Research Council; req, requirement; suppl, supplementation; TDN, total digestible nutrients; WW, weaning weight; YW, yearling weight.

up and down arrows represent the change in performance for offspring of lower plane of nutrition animals compared to control offspring.

[a] Diet = dietary treatment imposed on dams during gestation.
[b] Treatment = additional management imposed separate from diet.
[c] BW at 1-year of age or at prebreeding or at the end of the finishing period.
[d] Marbling score.
[e] Feed efficiency.
[f] Overall or final pregnancy rate.

that are grazing. However, this poses challenges with developmental programming studies due to the variation in grazing animal intake.[4] Grazing ruminants have an innate ability to compensate for nutritionally restricted environments. Although the forage may be nutritionally inadequate as determined by laboratory analysis, it is difficult to predict intake and diet selection during grazing. Supplementation does increase the nutritive value of the diet and can be assumed to improve performance. However, the ability for grazing ruminants to alter selectivity during grazing can decrease experimental treatment nutritive differences. Stalker and colleagues[5] and Martin and colleagues[6] reported the results from a 3-year study in which pregnant cows during late gestation grazed dormant range and received either 0.45 kg/d 42% crude protein (CP) cubes or no supplement. Masticate quality averaged across years was 5.4% CP and 50.1% total digestible nutrients (TDN) (dry matter basis). Although dry matter intake (DMI) was not directly measured it was estimated using the National Research Council (NRC) model.[7] These diets combined with supplement provided a difference in CP intake of 0.22 kg between treatments and TDN intake differed by 0.63 kg. There were no differences in heifer progeny birth BW and weaning weight (WW) but an increase in prebreeding BW was observed.[6] This translated to an increase in overall pregnancy rates and an increase in the number of heifer progeny that calved within the first 21 days of the calving season. However, Stalker and colleagues[5] reported an increase in steer WW but no difference in carcass quality (expressed as marbling score) across treatments. Interestingly, both treatments were considered deficient in net energy maintenance (NEm) (−0.45 vs −0.34 Mcal/d) and metabolizable protein (MP) (−102 vs −30 g/d).

Larson and colleagues[8] and Funston and colleagues[9] used a similar approach with protein supplementation but compared 2 different grazed forages. Using a 2-by-2 factorial arrangement of treatments, cows were assigned to native winter range or corn residue and either received (0.45 kg/d of a 28% CP supplement) or did not receive protein supplementation. A grazing system–supplementation interaction occurred, with a greater response to protein supplementation being observed for the native range group when compared with corn residue. This was despite that corn residue was of lower quality (5.2% CP and 52.7% TDN) than the rangeland (6.8% CP and 54.4% TDN). The corn residue treatment provided greater opportunity for selective grazing; therefore, protein supplementation was of little benefit to the subsequent progeny. This is supported by the notion that the 4 treatments in the current set of experiments provided 66%, 82%, 86%, and 103% of NRC protein requirements[7] for corn residue with no supplement, corn residue with supplement, native rangeland with no supplement, and native rangeland with supplement, respectively. When the investigators compared the main effects of grazing treatment, it was observed that corn residue progeny had greater birth BW for steers and not for heifers and WW was greater for both sexes. Interestingly, there was a forage–protein supplement interaction for heifer feed efficiency expressed as a gain-to-feed ratio. No differences were reported for native pasture treatments; however, heifers from dams that were not fed protein while grazing corn residue were more efficient than those from protein-supplemented dams. Overall, there were no differences in heifer reproduction or steer carcass quality as influenced by grazing system of the dam. Because of the variation in the basal diet provided to the cows during the third trimester, it is difficult to conclude that protein supplementation was responsible for alterations in progeny performance.

Mohrhauser and colleagues[10] and Taylor and colleagues[11] compared cows grazing versus drylot with the daily requirement supply restricted to 80% of requirements during midgestation in an effort to place cows in a positive or negative energy balance. Overal, no differences were observed in progeny growth performance characteristics. In this case, restriction of 80% may not have been severe enough to elicit a change in progeny response. It has been observed that ruminants subjected to intake restriction will reduce the nutrient passage rate from the rumen, which can increase ruminal degradability of nutrients.[12] Increases in ruminal degradability associated with decreased ruminal passage rate provides a greater residence time within the rumen and increases nutrient digestibility and supply to the animal. However, severe nutrient restriction (50% of requirement) reduces fetal fluid concentrations of alpha amino acids compared with animals receiving 100% of requirement.[13] Due to restructuring of placental tissues during restriction,[14] realimentation or refeeding increases supply to the fetal tissues.[15] In a natural setting, prolonged nutrient deprivation is rare and, in most cases, forage quality will increase, therefore mimicking a realimentation period, which may be partly responsible for the lack of differences when nutrient restriction is imposed during early gestation or midgestation.

Undernutrition

Livestock producers continually balance financial costs with providing a well-balanced diet. Nonetheless, mature animals are in a continual flux of gaining and losing weight. As previously stated, grazing ruminants can adapt behaviors to overcome nutritional stressors. However, there are times when the metabolism of the body must attempt to adapt to poor nutritional conditions; if it does not, productivity is hindered. The phenomenon of compensatory gain after growth restriction is an example of how dynamic the body can be to overcome nutritional deficiencies. The improved performance often observed with compensatory gain has been linked to a reduction in the net energy gain (NEg) requirement by approximately 18%, due in part to changes in body composition.[16] In addition, the metabolic hormones, such as insulin-like growth factor (IGF)-I and growth hormone, are altered such that when an animal is realimented to a higher plane of nutrition, growth rate is improved.[17] Likewise, the gastrointestinal tract and liver undergo changes in weight and cellularity during nutrient restriction and realimentation.[18] These all combine to provide the animal with the ability to overcome nutritional stress provided diet quality improves. In the pregnant animal, messenger RNA and protein expression of nutrient transporters in placental tissue is upregulated when ewes were nutrient restricted during early gestation to midgestation.[19] These physiologic responses indicate that the animal will adapt to nutrient restriction and progeny outcomes may not be observed.

The level at which an animal responds to nutrient restriction depends on the severity of the restriction. At this point, the literature does not indicate a specific level of restriction will initiate these changes. Therefore, it is difficult to ascertain if the differences observed in some experiments or lack thereof in others are due to inadequate level of nutrient restriction or due to the adaptive mechanisms used by the body. For livestock production, development of a greater understanding of these will assist in allocation of nutrients to livestock during key developmental windows. Specifically, knowledge of what type of nutrients can and cannot be restricted could allow formulation of rations that are cheaper, without negatively impacting animal productivity.

To delineate the effects of energy and protein on fetal programming, cattle were placed on 1 of 3 treatments: a well-fed group, restricted to 70% of NEm, and restricted and provided a supplement balanced to supply equal amounts of essential amino acids to the small intestine as the well-fed treatment during early gestation to midgestation.[20] Cow BW did not differ during early and midgestation until day 185 when all cows were switched to a common diet. Specifically, cows on the control and restricted plus protein were similar in BW and were greater than the nutrient-restricted cows. Interestingly, adipocyte diameter was greater for nutrient-restricted than for control or restricted plus protein treatments. Ovarian weight of heifer progeny was also reduced in nutrient-restricted treatments. Semitendinosus muscle (kg/hot carcass weight, percent) was reduced for the nutrient-restricted group and did not differ between the control and nutrient-restricted plus protein groups. This variation in tissue response indicates that certain tissues react to energy and protein deficits differently. This may explain the variation reported in **Table 1** across the various experiments.

Interpretation of data from maternal nutrition studies is difficult due to the myriad of factors that can influence postnatal performance of calves.[21] Nutritional treatments during pregnancy accounted for approximately 49.6% of the calf birthweight variation observed in the studies, whereas the remaining variation was influenced by postpartum BW of dam, sire breed, calf sex, birth day, and year. Additionally, when postpartum BW was fitted to statistical models, maternal nutrition did not affect calf birth weight, which illustrates the level at which the dam will conserve nutrient supply to the developing fetus to her own detriment. That being said, there are several experiments in which calf birth BW did not differ yet postnatal performance of the calf did differ between maternal nutritional treatments.[5,8,9,22–24]

Overnutrition

It is rare to find overfed livestock in a production setting; however, it is not unreasonable to expect greater performance in animals that are fed well above maintenance. Animal reproduction and growth is frequently observed to be greater in such a case. This of course can have negative ramifications as well. In humans, it has been well-established that children born to obese mothers have an increased risk of diabetes and other metabolic disease in adolescence and adulthood.[25] Additionally, Da Silva and colleagues[26] reported fetuses from adolescent ewes fed high amounts of a complete diet had reduced follicle numbers compared with ewes fed to gain 50 to 75 g/d through the first 100 days of gestation. However, it is not clear what the threshold would be regarding a positive or negative impact on progeny due to overnutrition.

Marques and colleagues[22] classified cattle body condition score (BCS) as adequate ($\geq$5.5 but $\leq$6.5, average BCS of 5.85) or inadequate ($\leq$4.75) at the beginning of gestation. Animals from the inadequate BCS group were randomly assigned to either maintain their current BCS or gain 1.5 BCS during the first, second, or third trimester, and to maintain that BCS until parturition. After calving, all cows were maintained similarly. Calf birth and weaning BW was similar between adequate and inadequate BCS. Likewise, calf birth and weaning BW did not differ when gestated by cows that gained 1.5 BCS during the first trimester compared with calves from adequate BCS cows. However, calves born to dams that gained 1.5 BCS during the second or third trimester had greater WW than adequate BCS calves. Calves from cows fed to maintain the inadequate BCS weaned at the same BW as those from the high and BCS gain in first trimester. This agrees with Mulliniks and colleagues,[27] who reported that steers from cows that gained or maintained BCS during gestation tended to have increased average daily gain (ADG) in the feedlot but carcass characteristics were not different. However, steers from cows that lost BCS and cows that were at a BCS of 4 during gestation had a greater percentage of steer calves that graded at choice or greater. Overall, this supports the notion that maintaining or gaining BCS is beneficial, and may indicate that energy is more influential than protein.

As research continues in the area of fetal programming, the identification of a specific nutrient that will provide the greatest impact on animal performance is needed. Micke and colleagues[23] fed either 240% or 70% of the daily protein requirements to beef cows during early gestation or midgestation. The result was 4 treatments that were high protein throughout early gestation and midgestation, low protein then high, high then low protein, or low protein for the duration of the experiment. Excessive protein supplementation during early gestation did not alter calf birth BW, whereas exposure during the second trimester increased calf birth weight. Weaning BW did not differ for any of the treatments. Male calves born to dams fed low protein during the first trimester had greater BW after weaning through the end of the experiment (657 days of age), whereas females did not differ. Maternal nutrition did not affect plasma IGF-I.

Shoup and colleagues[24,28] offered cows no supplement, low level of supplement (2.16 kg·cow^{-1} d^{-1} [per-cow-per-day]), or high level of supplement (8.61 kg·cow^{-1} d^{-1} [per-cow-per-day]) during late gestation. Supplement was 21.7% CP and 85.6% TDN on a DM basis. The resultant progeny were either early weaned (78 days of age) or normal weaned (186 days of age). Early wean BW was greater for supplemented groups compared with nonsupplemented controls and only differed by 5.5 kg. However, at the normal weaning time, steer BW did not differ. During the feeding and finishing period, growth performance, feed efficiency, and carcass quality did not differ across treatments. It should be noted that cow precalving BW (measured 49 days precalving) was greater for the high supplemented group compared with the no supplement and low supplement groups. This suggests that the no supplement group was not in a negative nutritional status, which is further supported by the overall lack of differences in reproductive performance across all treatments. It is not clear why calf BW differences were observed at the early wean time point but were short-lived. This could potentially be due to milk production differences for cows on the high level of supplement but cannot be confirmed because the investigators did not collect milk samples. Overall, the variation in nutritional status between the experimental treatments may have not been great enough to elicit responses similar to those reported previously.[5,6,8]

It is possible that the source of supplement could affect responses; specifically, ruminal degradability could influence metabolic markers. Ruminally degradable protein supports microbial CP synthesis, which supplies the animal with additional metabolizable protein. Whereas, ruminally undegradable protein will directly increase metabolizable protein supply. An increase in metabolizable protein supply has been reported to increase serum insulin production due to it being a glucogenic precursor.[29] Wilson and colleagues[30] provided beef cows rations that varied in ruminal degradability during late gestation. Treatments were designed to provide either a low (694 g/d) or high (975 g/d) amount of rumen degradable protein (RDP). Calf birth BW was greater for progeny gestated by cows fed the low RDP treatment. Weaning BW, final finished BW, and carcass traits did not differ between treatments. These results are supported by the work of Summers and colleagues[31,32] in which supplements that differed in ruminal degradability of protein and were fed during the third trimester to beef heifers did not influence any growth parameters or carcass characteristics of progeny. Although, it should be noted that, in these studies, pregnant heifers in the control group receiving no supplement were fed ad libitum grass hay, which resulted in animals being able to meet NE requirements.[31] Diets offered by Wilson and colleagues[30] did differ in energy content (TDN) but animals were fed at differing levels to provide similar total daily TDN intake. Therefore, supplemental ruminally degradable or undegradable protein may not have been offered at a level great enough to elicit a response by progeny. Although protein is often the most limiting nutrient on rangeland, it is difficult to delineate the impact of energy or protein in ruminants. This is because protein can be used for not only protein synthesis but as an energy source, as reported by Mulliniks and colleagues.[29] Long and colleagues[20] attempted to address this issue by providing a high rumen undegradable protein (RUP) supplement to normalize the intestinal supply of essential amino acids when cattle were limit fed. However, as reported previously, minimal effects were noted in progeny performance. It is possible that energy alone, irrespective of source (protein or carbohydrates) can be the major driver in the differences observed. This notion is supported by the various responses when cattle were managed for a greater BCS. During midgestation to late gestation, Wilson and colleagues[33] fed cows a diet that supplied 100% or 125% of TDN requirements. Researchers reported an increase in birth and weaning BW. However, no differences were observed in carcass quality.

Maternal Adaptation to Environmental Influences

Environmental influences can be attributed to manmade or management-related influences, as well as natural influences (eg, temperature, precipitation, day length). One hypothesis for altering performance based on environmental stimuli would be related to transgenerational programming, which results from environmental stimuli experienced by previous generations, effecting subsequent generations of offspring and grand-offspring.[34] Several studies report alterations in grandchild health in later life and lifespan when grandparents experience poor nutrition during gestation or early childhood.[35,36] Additional information regarding the influence of transgenerational programming on plants, animals, and insects has recently been reviewed.[34]

Vonnahme and colleagues,[37] in a 2-by-2 factorial study, investigated the influence of nutritional level and production environment on maternal and fetal growth, performance, and efficiency. Ewes came from 1 of 2 production environments. The first was a nomadic existence in which ewes were adapted over a 30-year period to an environment with limited nutritional supplementation and subsided mostly on high mountain pastures (Baggs). The second production environment was maintained in a relatively sedentary lifestyle, in which ewes consumed a diet that met or exceeded NRC requirements (SED). Additionally, ewes from each management system were fed 1 of 2 diets: 100% NRC recommendations (CON) or 50% NRC requirements (NR) beginning on day 28 of gestation through day 78. BCS and overall BW change remained relatively consistent during the 50-day feeding period for the CON-fed ewes from each group. However, differences in a ewe's ability to adapt to the NR diet were influenced by production environment. Ewes from the Baggs environment maintained BCS over the first 25 days before an approximate 1-point drop in overall condition (5.7 vs 4.9 ± 0.2) by day 78; whereas, SED ewes lost an average of 1.8 BCS during the 50-day period (5.4 vs 3.8 ± 0.2). Alterations in condition score are likely reflected in the loss of BW reported by the investigators. Sedate ewes fed the NR diet lost the greatest proportion of BW during the feeding period, suggesting this group may be more sensitive to nutrient restriction than the Baggs ewes, which were developed and selected for a production system with limited inputs.[37]

Fetal weight was similar among CON ewes and NR Baggs ewes regardless of fetal number (singleton vs twin). Additionally, fetal weights for NR SED ewes were decreased compared with all other treatment groups (**Table 2**). However, total placentome number was reduced for singleton pregnancy NR Baggs ewes compared with all other treatment groups. Placentome weight was greatest for CON SED ewes (1241 ± 89) with twin pregnancies and did not differ from NR Baggs ewes (1179 ± 145) with twin pregnancies.[37] Alterations in placentome number or weight could reflect the overall ability of the dam to transport nutrients to the offspring, thus altering fetal growth.

Additionally, Beard and colleagues[38] reported that calves born to cows experiencing low precipitation levels during early gestation had reduced birth and weaning BW compared with the counterparts gestated during average or wet years. However, calves born to cows experiencing low levels of precipitation in

Table 2
Influence of environment and nutritional status on ewe performance

Item[f]	SED[b]				Baggs[c]			
	CON[d]		NR[e]		CON[d]		NR[e]	
	Single	Twin	Single	Twin	Single	Twin	Single	Twin
Fetal weight (g)	309 ± 22a	307 ± 19a	235 ± 4a	215 ± 6a	283 ± 6a	260 ± 10a	285 ± 14a	273 ± 12a
Placentomes, (n)	86 ± 3a	84 ± 3a	78 ± 4a	81 ± 2a	93 ± 2a	93 ± 3a	59 ± 18a	79 ± 8a
Total placentome weight (g)	696 ± 29a	1241 ± 89a	821 ± 92a,c	936 ± 36c	729 ± 35a	1000 ± 15a	592 ± 123a	1179 ± 145a

a Within ewe type (Baggs or SED), row means with different superscripts differ ($P<.05$).
b Selected to a sedentary confinement-based management system.
c Selected to a nomadic extensive-based management system.
d Fed 100% NRC (1985) recommendations from gestational days 28 through 78.
e Fed 50% NRC (1985) recommendations from gestational d 28 through 78.
f Values for twin fetuses were first averaged, then this mean was used to generate group averages.
Adapted from Vonnahme KA, Hess BW, Nijland MJ, et al. Placentomal differentiation may compensate for maternal nutrient restriction in ewes adapted to harsh range conditions. J Anim Sci 2006;84(12):3451–9; with permission.

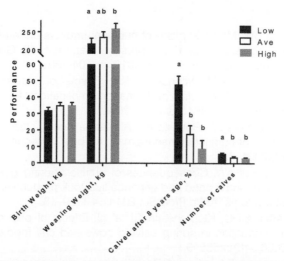

Fig. 1. Influence of precipitation level received during early gestation on female progeny performance. Data were collected over a 45-year period at the Chihuahuan Desert Rangeland Research Center. Based on average annual precipitation cows were classified as experience: low (black bars), ave (average, open bars), or high (gray bars) during early gestation, corresponding with the monsoon season. Within traits, means with different subscript letters differ ($P<.05$). (*Adapted from* Beard JK, Silver GA, Scholljegerdes EJ, et al. The effect of precipitation received during gestation on progeny performance in Bos indicus–influenced beef cattle. Paper presented at: American Society of Animal Science Western Section 2017; Fargo, ND, with permission.)

early gestation produced more calves and remained in the herd for a longer period of time compared with heifer calves gestated during average or high precipitation years (**Fig. 1**). Data from these studies and others may indicate the ability of livestock to adapt the environment and develop mechanisms to deliver nutrients to the offspring, thus programming for the potential environmental influences.

SUMMARY

Overall, there does not seem to be a consistent response in progeny outcomes with alterations in gestational nutrition of grazing livestock. This variation is likely attributed to the timing of supplementation and what key fetal physiologic systems are developed. Additionally, the grazing ruminant's innate ability to alter grazing behavior and ruminal fermentation characteristics are such that dietary deficiencies can be ameliorated to a certain extent. What does seem to be clear is that experiments that involve extreme differences between treatments, including nutrient restriction to around 50%, provide the most consistent progeny responses. Therefore, future work should continue to assess progeny outcomes, with an emphasis on monitoring overall dietary nutrient intake focused on energy and type of protein. Additionally, work is warranted in the area of how specific nutrients or molecules (eg, individual amino acids or metabolites) can affect progeny outcomes. Future work needs to continue to refine the understanding of how maternal nutrition can influence progeny outcomes, which will be extremely impactful to livestock producers.

REFERENCES

1. Caton JS, Hess BW. Maternal plane of nutrition: Impacts on fetal outcomes and postnatal offspring responses. Paper presented at: Proc. 4th Grazing Livestock Nurtition Conference. Estes Park, CO, 2010. p. 104-130.
2. Funston RN, Larson DM, Vonnahme KA. Effects of maternal nutrition on conceptus growth and offspring performance: implications for beef cattle production. J Anim Sci 2010;88(13 Suppl):E205-15.
3. Funston RN, Summers AF, Roberts AJ. Alpharma Beef Cattle Nutrition Symposium: implications of nutritional management for beef cow-calf systems. J Anim Sci 2012;90(7):2301-7.
4. Greenwood PL, Bell AW. Consequences of nutrition during gestation, and the challenge to better understand and enhance livestock productivity and efficiency in pastoral ecosystems. Anim Prod Sci 2014;54:1109-18.
5. Stalker LA, Adams DC, Klopfenstein TJ, et al. Effects of pre- and postpartum nutrition on reproduction in spring calving cows and calf feedlot performance. J Anim Sci 2006;84(9):2582-9.
6. Martin JL, Vonnahme KA, Adams DC, et al. Effects of dam nutrition on growth and reproductive performance of heifer calves. J Anim Sci 2007;85(3):841-7.
7. National Research Council. Nutrient requirements of beef cattle. 7th edition. Washington, DC: National Academy Press; 1996.
8. Larson DM, Martin JL, Adams DC, et al. Winter grazing system and supplementation during late gestation influence performance of beef cows and steer progeny. J Anim Sci 2009;87(3):1147-55.
9. Funston RN, Martin JL, Adams DC, et al. Winter grazing system and supplementation of beef cows during late gestation influence heifer progeny. J Anim Sci 2010;88(12):4094-101.
10. Mohrhauser DA, Taylor AR, Underwood KR, et al. The influence of maternal energy status during midgestation on beef offspring carcass characteristics and meat quality. J Anim Sci 2015;93(2):786-93.
11. Taylor AR, Mohrhauser DA, Prichard RH, et al. The influence of maternal energy status during midgestation on growth, cattle performance, and the immune response in the resultant beef progeny. Prof Anim Sci 2016;32:389-99.
12. Scholljegerdes EJ, Ludden PA, Hess BW. Effect of restricted forage intake on ruminal disappearance of bromegrass hay and a blood meal, feather meal, and fish meal supplement. J Anim Sci 2005;83(9):2146-50.
13. Kwon H, Ford SP, Bazer FW, et al. Maternal nutrient restriction reduces concentrations of amino acids and polyamines in ovine maternal and fetal plasma and fetal fluids. Biol Reprod 2004;71(3):901-8.
14. Gardner DS, Ward JW, Giussani DA, et al. The effect of a reversible period of adverse intrauterine conditions during late gestation on fetal and placental weight and placentome distribution in sheep. Placenta 2002;23(6):459-66.
15. Bell AW, Ehrhardt RA. Regulation of placental nutrient transport and implications for fetal growth. Nutr Res Rev 2002;15(2):211-30.
16. Carstens GE, Johnson DE, Ellenberger MA, et al. Physical and chemical components of the empty body during compensatory growth in beef steers. J Anim Sci 1991;69(8):3251-64.
17. Ellenberger MA, Johnson DE, Carstens GE, et al. Endocrine and metabolic changes during altered growth rates in beef cattle. J Anim Sci 1989;67(6):1446-54.

18. Sainz RD, Bentley BE. Visceral organ mass and cellularity in growth-restricted and refed beef steers. J Anim Sci 1997;75(5):1229–36.

19. Ma Y, Zhu MJ, Uthlaut AB, et al. Upregulation of growth signaling and nutrient transporters in cotyledons of early to midgestational nutrient restricted ewes. Placenta 2011;32(3):255–63.

20. Long NM, Tousley CB, Underwood KR, et al. Effects of early- to midgestational undernutrition with or without protein supplementation on offspring growth, carcass characteristics, and adipocyte size in beef cattle. J Anim Sci 2012; 90(1):197–206.

21. Robinson DL, Cafe LM, Greenwood PL. Meat Science and Muscle Biology Symposium: developmental programming in cattle: consequences for growth, efficiency, carcass, muscle, and beef quality characteristics. J Anim Sci 2013; 91(3):1428–42.

22. Marques RS, Cooke RF, Rodrigues MC, et al. Impacts of cow body condition score during gestation on weaning performance of the offspring. Livest Sci 2016;191:174–8.

23. Micke GC, Sullivan TM, Gatford KL, et al. Nutrient intake in the bovine during early and midgestation causes sex-specific changes in progeny plasma IGF-I, liveweight, height and carcass traits. Anim Reprod Sci 2010;121(3–4):208–17.

24. Shoup LM, Kloth AC, Wilson TB, et al. Prepartum supplement level and age at weaning: I. Effects on pre- and postpartum beef cow performance and calf performance through weaning. J Anim Sci 2015;93(10):4926–35.

25. Heerwagen MJ, Miller MR, Barbour LA, et al. Maternal obesity and fetal metabolic programming: a fertile epigenetic soil. Am J Physiol Regul Integr Comp Physiol 2010;299(3):R711–22.

26. Da Silva P, Aitken RP, Rhind SM, et al. Impact of maternal nutrition during pregnancy on pituitary gonadotrophin gene expression and ovarian development in growth-restricted and normally grown late gestation sheep fetuses. Reproduction 2002;123(6):769–77.

27. Mulliniks JT, Sawyer JE, Harrelson FW, et al. Effect of late gestation bodyweight change and condition score on progeny feedlot performance. Anim Prod Sci 2016;56:1998–2003.

28. Shoup LM, Wilson TB, Gonzalez-Pena D, et al. Beef cow prepartum supplement level and age at weaning: II. Effects of developmental programming on performance and carcass composition of steer progeny. J Anim Sci 2015;93(10): 4936–47.

29. Mulliniks JT, Cox SH, Kemp ME, et al. Protein and glucogenic precursor supplementation: a nutritional strategy to increase reproductive and economic output. J Anim Sci 2011;89(10):3334–43.

30. Wilson TB, Faulkner DB, Shike DW. Influence of late gestation drylot rations differing in protein degradability and fat content on beef cow and subsequent calf performance. J Anim Sci 2015;93(12):5819–28.

31. Summers AF, Meyer TL, Funston RN. Impact of supplemental protein source offered to primiparous heifers during gestation on I. Average daily gain, feed intake, calf birth body weight, and rebreeding in pregnant beef heifers. J Anim Sci 2015;93(4):1865–70.

32. Summers AF, Blair AD, Funston RN. Impact of supplemental protein source offered to primiparous heifers during gestation on II. Progeny performance and carcass characteristics. J Anim Sci 2015;93(4):1871–80.

33. Wilson TB, Faulkner DB, Shike DW. Influence of prepartum dietary energy on beef cow performance and calf growth and carcass characteristics. Livest Sci 2016; 184:21–7.

34. Burton T, Metcalfe NB. Can environmental conditions experienced in early life influence future generations? Proc Biol Sci 2014;281(1785):20140311.

35. Painter RC, Osmond C, Gluckman P, et al. Transgenerational effects of prenatal exposure to the Dutch famine on neonatal adiposity and health in later life. BJOG 2008;115(10):1243–9.

36. Kaati G, Bygren LO, Pembrey M, et al. Transgenerational response to nutrition, early life circumstances and longevity. Eur J Hum Genet 2007;15(7):784–90.

37. Vonnahme KA, Hess BW, Nijland MJ, et al. Placentomal differentiation may compensate for maternal nutrient restriction in ewes adapted to harsh range conditions. J Anim Sci 2006;84(12):3451–9.

38. Beard JK, Silver GA, Scholljegerdes EJ, et al. The effect of precipitation received during gestation on progeny performance in Bos indicus–influenced beef cattle. Paper presented at: American Society of Animal Science Western Section. Fargo, ND, 2017.

39. Bohnert DW, Stalker LA, Mills RR, et al. Late gestation supplementation of beef cows differing in body condition score: effects on cow and calf performance. J Anim Sci 2013;91(11):5485–91.

40. Long NM, George LA, Uthlaut AB, et al. Maternal obesity and increased nutrient intake before and during gestation in the ewe results in altered growth, adiposity, and glucose tolerance in adult offspring. J Anim Sci 2010;88(11):3546–53.

41. Long NM, Prado-Cooper MJ, Krehbiel, et al. Effects of nutrient restriction of bovine dams during early gestation on postnatal growth, carcass and organ characteristics, and gene expression in adipose tissue and muscle. J Anim Sci 2010; 88(10):3251–61.

42. Marques RS, Cooke RF, Rodrigues MC, et al. Effects of organic or inorganic cobalt, copper, manganese, and zinc supplementation to late-gestating beef cows on productive and physiological responses of the offspring. J Anim Sci 2016; 94(3):1215–26.

43. Shoup LM, Miller LM, Srinivasan M, et al. Effects of cows grazing toxic endophyte-infected tall fescue or novel endophyte-infected tall fescue in late gestation on cow performance, reproduction, and progeny growth performance and carcass characteristics. J Anim Sci 2016;94(12):5105–13.

44. Wilson TB, Long NM, Faulkner DB, et al. Influence of excessive dietary protein intake during late gestation on drylot beef cow performance and progeny growth, carcass characteristics, and plasma glucose and insulin concentrations. J Anim Sci 2016;94(5):2035–46.

Developmental Programming in a Beef Production System

Devin Broadhead, BS[a], J. Travis Mulliniks, PhD[b],
Rick N. Funston, PhD[c],*

KEYWORDS

- Beef cattle • Fetal programming • Production systems • Protein supplementation

KEY POINTS

- Initiation of developmental programming occurs during the early stages of gestation.
- Several factors influence developmental programming, including environment, grazing management, supplement type and amount, and long-term management within an environment.
- Prepartum protein supplementation can increase subsequent pregnancy rates, progeny weaning weight, and progeny health.
- Production environment during gestation can influence progeny heifer growth and reproductive performance.

INTRODUCTION

Beef production is a complex, integrated system involving environmental influences and management decisions from conception to end product, whether it be a carcass or a breeding female. Beef production systems balance nutritional decisions based on economic and production outputs. Several factors influence nutritional management decisions, such as forage quality and quantity, cow condition, production goals, labor availability, and cost. Grazing dormant pasture can minimize production costs significantly but can also affect cow maintenance, fetal development, and future calf performance. In profit models, increasing feed amounts per cow to meet or exceed cow requirements did not increase production or calving profits but did increase costs.[1]

Disclosure Statement: The authors have nothing to disclose.
[a] Agricultural Economics, University of Nebraska, West Central Research and Extension Center, 402 West State Farm Road, North Platte, NE 69101, USA; [b] Beef Production Systems, University of Nebraska, West Central Research and Extension Center, 402 West State Farm Road, North Platte, NE 69101, USA; [c] University of Nebraska, West Central Research and Extension Center, 402 West State Farm Road, North Platte, NE 69101, USA
* Corresponding author.
E-mail address: rick.funston@unl.edu

Vet Clin Food Anim 35 (2019) 379–390
https://doi.org/10.1016/j.cvfa.2019.02.011
0749-0720/19/© 2019 Elsevier Inc. All rights reserved.

Targeting supplementation to critical physiologic periods may provide an opportunity to reduce production costs and positively affect developmental programming. Altering grazing systems and management, and supplement timing and type, can improve nutrient utilization in an attempt to improve production efficiency. In many cases, these strategies may affect a cow minimally but influence production traits throughout the life of her calves. This is considered developmental programming: the concept that the in utero environment during critical periods of fetal development affects the offspring throughout its lifetime. Developmental programming can either positively or negatively affect the future production of the subsequent offspring. This article discusses developmental programming during midgestation and late gestation in a beef production system.

PRODUCTION ENVIRONMENTS AND FETAL PROGRAMMING

Matching nutrient requirements with nutrient availability optimizes production efficiency. Forage systems and livestock production are intertwined. During the production cycle for most beef producers in the western United States, rangeland forage is dormant during times of significant biological energy demand (gestation, parturition, and lactation). Depending on season of calving, gestating cows often graze in production systems that do not meet their nutrient requirements. If dietary nutrient intake does not meet nutrient requirements, body tissue reserves (both lean and adipose tissue) will be mobilized to balance the deficiency. In most forage-based production systems, forage quality and quantity is highly dynamic and depends on environmental conditions (ie, timing and amount of rainfall) and management. For instance, Nebraska Sandhills upland native range can range from 6.2% to 12.4% crude protein (CP) with corresponding total digestible nutrient values of 49.9% to 64.8% during the year.[2] Seasonal variation in forage production challenges beef producers. Diverse production systems using pastures, harvested forages, and crop residues have evolved in different regions of the United States in response to soil and climate, competing requirements for land and water resources, and the relative cost and availability of feed grains.[3] Consequently, there is a need to understand how different environments and forage systems affect the entire production system from conception to slaughter.

GESTATIONAL SUPPLEMENTATION OVERVIEW

Nutritional management may not only affect maintenance, growth, or production in lactating or gestating cows but it can also influence fetal growth and subsequent postnatal performance. Undernutrition during gestation causes suboptimal conditions in the maternal uterine environment, which may positively or negatively influence the development of fetal organs and tissues and lead to lifetime impacts on progeny performance. Inadequate placental size or function can further complicate the influence of maternal nutrition on fetal development. For example, well-fed dams may still have an undernourished fetus because placental development or capacity is not adequate to meet fetal demands.[4,5] However, the fetus may have a natural protection against prepartum undernutrition of the dam by mobilizing maternal body reserves.[6] Even when the dam is undernourished, the maternal and placental systems may compensate so that fetal malnutrition is minimal.[6,7] Proper nutritional management during gestation is still a priority to improve subsequent progeny's performance and health. Timing of nutritional restriction can also affect a developing fetus. Owing to the minimal nutrient requirements of the fetus during early gestation in many environments, nutrition restriction during this time has historically been considered to have little to minimal negative impact on fetal growth. However, during fetal development from midgestation to late gestation, critical events for normal conceptus development occur, including fetal organogenesis and placental development.[8] Manipulating maternal nutrition during specific periods of gestation can result in the programming of fetal and postnatal development of the subsequent progeny. Increased rate of growth of the developing fetus during midgestation to late gestation places more metabolic demand on the cow. Because growth predominates during the latter half of gestation and is of a lower priority for nutrient partitioning in the fetus, suboptimal maternal nutrition at this stage can negatively affect fetal growth and muscle development.

Environmental conditions and long-term management can affect how livestock respond to environmental stress and nutrient restriction. Comparing long-term (adapted over 30 years) management in farm sheep flocks, maternal undernutrition in gestating ewes from nutrient-restricted environments did not affect fetal growth, plasma glucose concentrations,[9] or amino acid concentrations.[10] These studies imply the dam and fetus may have the ability to provide a natural adjustment against nutrient restrictions when livestock are managed long-term in their environment. Research with fish gives insight into long-term management in highly variable, harsh environments and how they cope with those stressors. Transgenerational acclimation in fish illustrates how single-generation studies may underestimate the potential of cattle to cope and adapt.[11] Therefore, in many production settings, the developmental programming response in nutrient-restricted environments may positively affect developing animals better adapted and resilient in those environmental conditions.

IMPACT OF GESTATIONAL NUTRITION ON COW PERFORMANCE

During certain times in the production cycle, nutrient and forage availability may be insufficient to meet cow requirements in some environments. Under these conditions, a reduced energy intake may occur, possibly leading to negative energy balance. Supplements can be provided to minimize the body tissue mobilized to meet maintenance and production requirements. Periods of insufficient nutrient intake are often followed by compensatory gain, which may have a limited impact on mature breeding animals. Research has indicated management strategies can bring about moderate stages of feed restriction and realimentation during periods of poor nutrient availability to improve nutrient utilization.[12,13] For instance, in a 7-year study, Mulliniks and colleagues[14] reported overall pregnancy rates were greater in cows either losing or maintaining weight during late gestation compared with cows gaining weight. Although weight change differences were not reported up to and through breeding, this improved reproductive performance may be attributed to a decrease in nutrient requirements in cows losing weight during late gestation and an overall increase in nutrient utilization postpartum.

Multiple studies have resulted in no differences in reproductive efficiency between supplementation and no supplementation during late gestation. These results indicate prepartum nutrition in mature cows may have less of a role in subsequent reproductive performance and more influence on fetal growth and subsequent progeny performance. At the University of Nebraska Gudmundsen Sandhills Laboratory, an ongoing meta-analysis of 15 years of research on protein supplementation during late gestation is being conducted to determine the influence of protein supplementation on cow–calf performance. Contrary to other studies, this meta-analysis indicates that protein supplement offered to cows grazing winter range increases subsequent pregnancy rates of gestating dams by 3% points compared with nonsupplemented cows. However, supplementation has not influenced cow prepartum weight change or body condition score during supplementation. Protein supplementation has been shown to increase cow weight gain while grazing low-quality dormant forage.[15] However, results from previous research evaluating prepartum supplementation effects on cow performance (**Table 1**) have varied greatly and been largely inconclusive.[16–18] This may be due to differences in amount and type of protein fed, total dietary protein intake, environmental conditions, nutrient use efficiency of the cowherd, and previous long-term management of the cows.

IMPACT OF GESTATIONAL NUTRITION ON FEMALE PROGENY PERFORMANCE

Data from 4 Nebraska studies that evaluated the effect of prepartum nutrition on heifer progeny performance are reported in **Table 2**. Maternal nutrition may influence subsequent heifer lifetime productivity in the cowherd. In addition, nutritional management as early as midgestation can affect organ development. In an early gestation to midgestation study,[19] cows were fed either 70% or 100% of their nutrient requirements from day 45 to 185 of gestation, and then all cows were fed to nutrient requirements from day 185 of gestation until calving. Although progeny birth and weaning weights were similar, heifers born to cows fed at 70% did have smaller ovaries and luteal tissue. This indicates midgestation nutrition can play a role in future reproductive performance of heifer progeny. In the Nebraska Sandhills, May-calving cows may experience nutrient restriction starting during midgestation. Lansford[20] evaluated progeny performance from cows grazing either native range or subirrigated meadow, with and without protein supplementation, during midgestation. Regardless of grazing treatment, protein supplementation during midgestation increased heifer progeny 205-day adjusted weaning weight compared with nonsupplemented dams. However, overall heifer pregnancy rates and timing of conception were not influenced by dam supplementation.

Warner and colleagues[21] reported no differences in pregnancy rates for heifers from dams grazing corn residue during late gestation with or without receiving protein supplement. Similarly, Funston and colleagues[8] reported protein supplementation to cows grazing corn residue during late gestation did not affect subsequent heifer fertility; however, there was a tendency for increased heifer pregnancy rates if heifers were born to cows supplemented on winter range compared with those nonsupplemented on winter range. Corah and colleagues[22] reported age at puberty of heifer progeny from energy-restricted primiparous dams was increased 19 days; however, the subsequent pregnancy rate was not measured. Dam nutrition within this study[22] did not affect heifer birth date or weight. Protein supplementation during late gestation tended to increase the subsequent weaning weight of heifer calves and increased the adjusted 205-day weight.[23] In addition, prebreeding and pregnancy diagnosis weights were greater for heifers from protein-supplemented dams than heifers from nonsupplemented dams.[23] Average daily gain between weaning and beginning of the first breeding season for heifers was not affected by dam treatment for 2 years out of a 3-year study by Martin and colleagues.[23] A study by Cushman and colleagues[24] examined how nutrient restriction to mature cows during the second and third trimester affected daughter growth and reproductive performance. These investigators reported no negative impact on growth rates, age at puberty, or antral follicle counts on heifer progeny. However, Martin and colleagues[23] reported a 28% increase in percentage of heifers calving in the first 21 days of the calving season from protein-supplemented dams compared with nonsupplemented dams. In contrast, Funston and colleagues[8] and Lansford[20] reported no difference in the proportion of heifers calving in the first 21 days. In agreement, Broadhead and colleagues,[25] using 15 years

Table 1
Effect of no supplementation versus prepartum protein supplementation while grazing dormant, low-quality, native range on cow performance and subsequent reproductive performance

Item	Stalker and colleagues[16–18]		Larson and colleagues[18]		Mulliniks and colleagues[19]		Broadhead and colleagues[25]	
	NS	SUP	NS	SUP	NS	SUP	NS	SUP
BW Change (kg)								
Prepartum	−29[a]	1[a]	—	—	−14[a]	2[a]	—	—
Postpartum	14	12	—	—	—	—	—	—
Body Condition Score Change								
Prepartum	−0.65[a]	−0.10[a]	—	—	−0.5[a]	0.0[a]	—	—
Postpartum	0.30	0.25	—	—	—	—	—	—
Calving Date (d)	85	88	89	83	—	—	82	82
Calved in first 21 d (%)	71	70	62	83	—	—	83	85
Pregnancy rate (%)	90	93	94	96	94	94	90[a]	93[a]

Abbreviations: BW, body weight; NS, no supplementation; SUP, supplementation.
[a] Means within a study with different superscripts differ (*P*<.05).

Table 2
Effect of no supplementation versus prepartum protein supplementation to dams while grazing dormant, low-quality, native range on heifer progeny performance

Item	Martin and colleagues,[23] 2007		Funston and colleagues,[8] 2010		Lansford,[20] 2018		Broadhead and colleagues[25]	
	NS	SUP	NS	SUP	NS	SUP	NS	SUP
Birthweight, kg	35	36	35	35	32	32	34	34
Adjusted 205-d Weight	218[a]	226[a]	213	217	187[a]	194[a]	220	224
Age at Puberty (d)	334	339	366	352	—	—	—	—
Puberty Status (%)	—	—	—	—	75	75	62	65
Prebreeding Weight (kg)	266	276	317	323	316	317	336	332
Pregnancy Diagnosis Weight (kg)	386	400	364	368	399	408	375	384
Pregnant (%)	80[a]	93[a]	80	90	82	86	90	90
Calved in First 21 d (%)	49[a]	77[a]	85	77	76	78	70	74

[a] Means within a study with different superscripts differ ($P<.05$).

of data, illustrated that heifer performance (body weight and reproductive performance) is not different from heifer progeny born from nonsupplemented and protein-supplemented dams during late gestation. In a long-term retrospective study, Beard and colleagues[26] determined that precipitation levels (ie, drought, average, or high rainfall years) during key fetal development periods affected progeny performance. Although drought conditions resulted in decreased heifer body weight at birth and weaning, heifer progeny experiencing drought in utero had increased lifetime retention and productivity in arid rangelands. Increased retention may have been due to increased adaptive capacity to environmental stressors in limited nutrient environments for offspring experiencing nutrient restriction in utero. Furthermore, increasing nutrient input during key physiologic periods may imprint progeny to require a greater level of nutrients to be reproductively competent in more arid environments.

IMPACT OF GESTATIONAL NUTRITION ON STEER PROGENY PERFORMANCE

Data from 5 late-gestation studies evaluating the influence of dam protein supplementation on steer progeny weaning and postweaning performance are reported in **Table 3**. In the Nebraska Sandhills, Lansford[20] illustrated protein supplementation during midgestation on dormant subirrigated meadow or native upland range did not affect calf growth from birth through weaning. In addition, midgestation protein supplementation did not influence feedlot average daily gain, hot carcass weight, twelfth rib fat thickness, or yield grade. Underwood and colleagues[27] studied the growth performance of steers born from dams that grazed either low-quality native range (6% CP) or high-quality irrigated pasture (11% CP) during midgestation. In contrast to the results of the previous study, weaning and carcass weights were reduced for steer progeny from cows that grazed low-quality native range pastures compared with steers from dams that grazed higher quality irrigated pastures during midgestation. Munoz and colleagues[28] evaluated how nutrient restriction during early pregnancy or midpregnancy affected lamb performance from birth to weaning. From conception to day 39 of gestation, these investigators fed diets that were deficient (60%), adequate (100%), or in excess (200%) of predicted metabolizable energy for maintenance. From day 40 to 90 of gestation, diets were deficient (80%) or in excess (140%) of their predicted metabolizable energy for maintenance. All ewes were fed at maintenance levels after day 90 of gestation. These researchers reported lambs from ewes fed a restricted diet in early pregnancy were born heavier, had higher immunoglobulin (Ig)G levels 24 hours after birth, and had a lower mortality rate at weaning than lambs from the adequate or excessive dams.

Stalker and colleagues[16] investigated how prepartum and postpartum nutrition affected calf growth and feedlot performance. Supplemental treatments included a 42% CP supplement at 0.45 kg/d or no supplement to cows grazing native range during late gestation. Calves from supplemented dams gained more and were heavier at weaning compared with calves from nonsupplemented cows. However, feedlot performance (average daily gain, feed efficiency, and dry matter intake) was similar for both groups of steer progeny, concluding that supplemental feeding to the dam may not influence steer progeny postweaning feedlot performance. In a second study conducted by Stalker and colleagues,[29] steers from supplemented dams had greater preweaning and postweaning gains compared with steers from nonsupplemented dams. However, Larson and colleagues[17] demonstrated dam nutrition did affect calf birth weight and early gains, and this difference persisted through weaning and slaughter. Steers from supplemented dams tended to gain more after placement in

Table 3
Effect of no supplementation versus prepartum protein supplementation to dams while grazing dormant, low-quality, native range on steer progeny performance

Item	Stalker and colleagues[29]		Stalker and colleagues[16]		Larson and colleagues[17] 2009		Mulliniks and colleagues[18] 2012		Broadhead and colleagues[25] (unpublished meta-analysis)	
	NS	SUP	NS	SUP	NS	SUP	NS	SUP	NS	SUP
Weaning BW (kg)	200[a]	210[a]	211[a]	218[a]	223[a]	241[a]	253	253	221[a]	228[a]
DMI (kg/d)	11.15[a]	12.05[a]	8.48	8.53	8.94	9.19	—	—	—	—
ADG (kg/d)	1.60	1.68	1.57	1.56	1.66	1.70	1.38	1.46	—	—
F:G	6.97	7.19	5.41	5.46	5.37	5.38	—	—	—	—
HCW (kg)	347[a]	365[a]	363	369	364[a]	372[a]	322	323	374	371
Choice (%)	—	—	85	96	71	86	—	—	—	—
Marbling Score	449	461	467	479	444[a]	493[a]	487	487	471	480

Abbreviations: ADG, average daily gain; DMI, dry matter intake; F:G, feed to gain ratio; HCW, hot carcass weight.
[a] Means within a study with different superscripts differ (*P*<.05).

the feedlot compared with steers from nonsupplemented dams. However, even with the tendency toward greater average daily gain and feed consumption on a per pen basis, overall gain efficiency was not different, similar to the results from Stalker and colleagues.[16] The unpublished, ongoing meta-analysis previously mentioned shows a 7 kg increase in weaning weight of calves from protein-supplemented dams compared with calves from nonsupplemented dams during late gestation. However, feedlot performance and carcass characteristics were not influenced by dam supplementation during late gestation. The response to protein supplementation during late gestation on steer weaning weight and carcass weight has been inconsistent. Studies that have reported an increase in weaning weight from dam supplementation have illustrated an increase in weight that continues to the carcass.[17,29] Other studies have shown no differences in feedlot performance or carcass characteristics between progeny from supplemented and nonsupplemented dams during late gestation.[16,18,30,31] Reasons for these varied results could be due to differences in long-term herd management, environmental conditions, genetic makeup of the cowherd, metabolic efficiency, and ability to adapt to environmental conditions.

IMPACT OF GESTATIONAL NUTRITION ON PROGENY HEALTH

In addition to influencing calf growth, undernutrition of gestating cows has been illustrated to reduce passive immunity.[32,33] Immune function is critical for calf health, which is directly correlated to feedlot performance, carcass value, and profitability. Blecha and colleagues[32] reviewed the effect of prepartum protein restriction in the last 100 days of gestation on IgG content in the blood and absorption of colostral whey and IgG by the neonatal calf. These investigators found no difference in immunoglobin concentrations in the serum or colostrum of the cow when fed different levels of protein. However, IgG absorption by the calf after birth increased as protein levels increased in the dam diet. This indicates calves from cows consuming low levels of protein might have decreased passive immunity transfer. Hough and colleagues[34] also reported that nutritional restriction during late gestation affected passive immunity in beef cattle. In this study, the restricted diet was 57% of NRC (National Research Council Nutrient Requirements for Beef Cattle)[4] requirements and the control diet was 100% of the NRC[4] requirements for both protein and energy. It should be noted that in production settings, livestock may never experience as severe a restriction as that of the Hough and colleagues[34] study. Nevertheless, serum IgG concentrations were not affected by prepartum nutritional management, suggesting the calves' ability to absorb IgG was not altered by maternal nutrient restriction.

Several studies have linked prepartum nutrition to subsequent calf health postweaning. Studies from New Mexico indicate prepartum supplementation strategy may not influence calf weaning weight or feedlot performance.[18,30] However, investigators reported that steer progeny born from dams provided a high rumen undegradable protein supplement were treated less for sickness and had decreased feedlot costs, whereas no differences in sickness between steer progeny from dams fed rumen degradable protein or no protein supplement occurred. This implies certain nutrient or ingredient formulations for range prepartum supplements may positively affect calf health and performance. Therefore, correctly managing the maternal diet during gestation may provide an opportunity to reduce sickness in the subsequent offspring during the feedlot phase. Reducing the occurrence of sickness and ensuing medical treatments improves feedlot profitability. Galyean[35] reported calves treated once for disease returned $40.62 less, calves treated twice returned $58.35 less, and calves treated 3 or more times returned $291.93 less compared with calves not treated.

SUMMARY

Management of maternal diet throughout gestation will ensure adequate nutrient transfer to the fetus. Maternal nutrition has been reported to influence fetal organ development, muscle development, postnatal calf performance, carcass characteristics, and reproduction. Responses to prepartum nutrition have been inconstant due to the highly variable nature of environmental conditions and management in beef production systems. However, prepartum supplementation, particularly high rumen, undegradable protein supplements, has shown positive impacts on subsequent progeny performance preweaning and postweaning.

REFERENCES

1. Ramsey R, Doye D, Ward C, et al. Factors affecting beef cow-herd costs, production, and profits. J Agric Appl Econ 2005;37:91–9.
2. Mulliniks JT, Adams DC. 2019. Evaluation of lactation demands on nutrient balance in two calving seasons in range cows grazing Sandhills upland range. Pages 18-20 in Univ. Nebraska Beef Report. Agric. Res. Devi., UNL Cooperative Extension, Lincoln, NE.
3. Reid RL, Klopfenstein TJ. Forage and crop residues: quality evaluation and systems of utilization. J Anim Sci 1983;57:534–62.
4. NRC. Nutrient requirements of beef cattle. 7th rev. Washington, DC: Natl. Acad. Press; 2000.
5. Martin GS, Carstens GE, Taylor TL, et al. Prepartum protein restriction does not alter norepinephrine-induced thermogenesis or brown adipose tissue function in newborn calves. J Nutr 1997;127:1929–37.
6. Bassett JM. Nutrition of the conceptus: aspects of its regulation. Proc Nutr Soc 1986;45:1–10.
7. Bassett JM. Current perspectives on placental development and its integration with fetal growth. Proc Nutr Soc 1991;50:311–9.
8. Funston RN, Larson DM, Vonnahme KA. Effects of maternal nutrition on conceptus growth and offspring performance: implications for beef cattle production. J Anim Sci 2010;88(Suppl):E205–15.
9. Vonnahme KA, Hess BW, Nijland MJ, et al. Placentomal differentiation may compensate for maternal nutrient restriction in ewes adapted to harsh range conditions. J Anim Sci 2006;84:3451–9.
10. Jobgen WS, Ford SP, Jobgen SC, et al. Baggs ewes adapt to maternal undernutrition and maintain conceptus growth by maintaining fetal plasma concentrations of amino acids. J Anim Sci 2008;86:820–6.
11. Donelson JM, Munday PL, McCormick MI, et al. Rapid transgenerational acclimation of a tropical reef fish to climate change. Nat Clim Chang 2012;2:30–2.
12. Freetly HC, Nienaber JA, Brown-Brandl T. Partitioning of energy in pregnant beef cows during nutritionally induced body weight fluctuation. J Anim Sci 2008;86:370–7.
13. Freetly HC, Nienaber JA. Efficiency of energy and nitrogen loss and gain in mature cows. J Anim Sci 1998;76:896–905.
14. Mulliniks JT, Sawyer JE, Harrelson FW, et al. Effect of late gestation bodyweight change and condition score on progeny feedlot performance. Anim Prod Sci 2016;56:1998–2003.
15. Clanton DC, Zimmerman DR. Symposium on pasture methods for maximum production of beef cattle: Protein and energy requirements for female beef cattle. J Anim Sci 1970;30:122.

16. Stalker LA, Adams DC, Klopfenstein TJ, et al. Effects of pre- and postpartum nutrition on reproduction in spring calving cows and calf feedlot performance. J Anim Sci 2006;84:2582–9.

17. Larson DM, Martin JL, Adams DC, et al. Winter grazing system and supplementation during late gestation influence performance of beef cows and steer progeny. J Anim Sci 2009;87:1147–55.

18. Mulliniks JT, Sawyer JE, Mathis CP, et al. Winter protein management during late gestation alters range cow and steer progeny performance. J Anim Sci 2012;90: 5099–106.

19. Long NM, Tousley CB, Underwood KR, et al. Effects of Early- to Mid-Gestational Undernutrition with or without Protein Supplementation on Offspring Growth, Carcass Characteristics, and Adipocyte Size in Beef Cattle. J Anim Sci 2012; 90:197–206.

20. Lansford AC. Supplementation and reproductive strategies for beef females as part of a May-calving herd in the Nebraska Sandhills. Master's thesis. Lincoln (NE): Univ of Nebraska; 2018.

21. Warner JM, Martin JL, Hall ZC, et al. The effects of supplementing beef cows grazing cornstalk residue with a dried distillers grain based cube on cow and calf performance. Prof Anim Sci 2011;27:540–6.

22. Corah LR, Dunn TG, Kalthenbach CC. Influence of prepartum nutrition on the reproductive performance of beef females and the performance of their progeny. J Anim Sci 1975;41:819–24.

23. Martin JL, Vonnahme KA, Adams DC, et al. Effects of dam nutrition on growth and reproductive performance of heifer calves. J Anim Sci 2007;85:841–7.

24. Cushman RA, McNeel AK, Freetly HC. The impact of cow nutrient status during the second and third trimesters on age at puberty, antral follicle count, and fertility of daughters. Livest Sci 2014;162:252–8.

25. Broadhead DL. Effects of late gestation supplementation and fetal programming methods on a spring calving beef herd in the Nebraska Sandhills. Master's Thesis. Lincoln (NE): Univ of Nebraska; 2019. in press.

26. Beard JK, Silver GA, Scholljegerdes EJ, et al. The effect of precipitation received during gestation on progeny performance in Bos indicus influenced beef cattle. Trans Anim Sci 2019. https://doi.org/10.1093/tas/txy139.

27. Underwood KR, Tong JF, Price PL, et al. Nutrition during mid to late gestation affects growth, adipose tissue deposition and tenderness in cross-bred beef steers. Meat Sci 2010;86:588–93.

28. Munoz C, Carson AF, McCoy MA, et al. Nutritional status of adult ewes during early and mid-pregnancy. 1. Effects of plane of nutrition on ewe reproduction and offspring performance to weaning. Animal 2008;2:52–63.

29. Stalker LA, Ciminski LA, Adams DC, et al. Effects of weaning date and prepartum protein supplementation on cow performance and calf growth. Rangeland Ecol Manage 2007;60:578–87.

30. Mulliniks JT, Mathis CP, Cox SH, et al. Supplementation strategy during late gestation alters steer progeny health in the feedlot without affecting cow performance. Anim Feed Sci Technol 2013;185:126–32.

31. Broadhead DL, Stalker LA, Musgrave JA, et al. Methods to increase productivity of spring calving production systems in the Nebraska Sandhills. Proc West Sec Am Soc Anim Sci 2016;67:17–9.

32. Blecha F, Bull RC, Olson DP, et al. Effects of prepartum protein restriction in the beef cow on immunoglobin content in blood and colostral whey and subsequent immunoglobin absorption by the neonatal calf. J Anim Sci 1981;53:1174–80.

33. Bellows RA, Short RE. Effects of precalving feed level on birth weight, calving difficulty and subsequent fertility. J Anim Sci 1978;46:1522–8.
34. Hough RL, McCarthy FD, Kent HD, et al. Influence of nutritional restriction during late gestation on production measures and passive immunity in beef cattle. J Anim Sci 1990;68:2622–7.
35. Galyean ML. Recent advances in management of highly stressed, newly received feedlot cattle. J Anim Sci 2006;85:823–40.

Printed and bound by CPI Group (UK) Ltd, Croydon, CR0 4YY

03/10/2024

01040403-0009